The Official
Body Control Pilates®
Manual

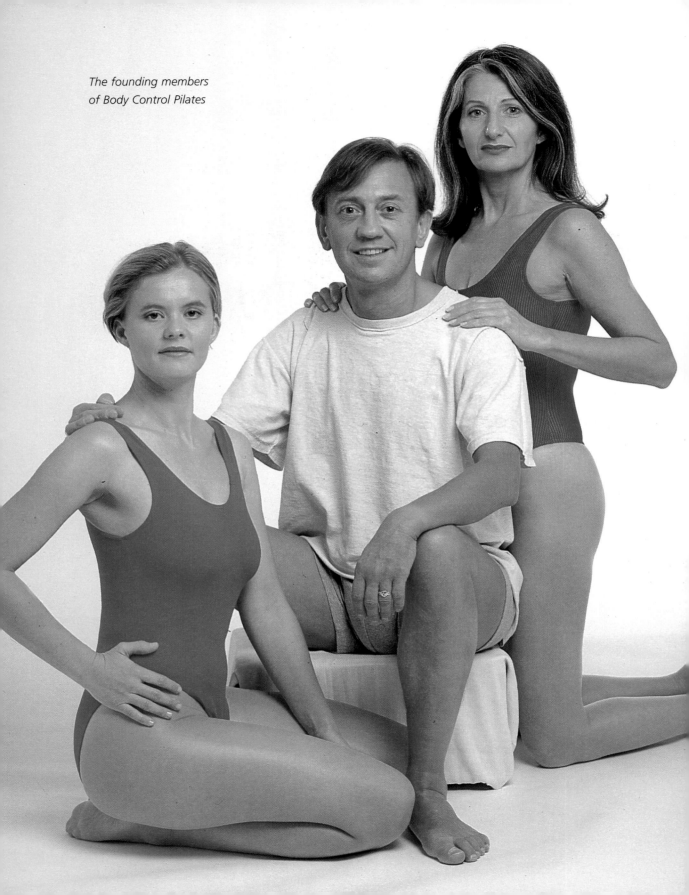

The Official
Body Control Pilates®
Manual

Lynne Robinson, Helge Fisher,
Jacqueline Knox MCSP SRP and Gordon Thomson

TED SMART

First published 2000 by Macmillan
an imprint of Macmillan Publishers Ltd
25 Eccleston Place, London SW1W 9NF
Oxford and Basingstoke
Associated companies throughout the world
www.macmillan.co.uk

This edition printed for The Book People 2001
Hallwood Avenue, Haydock, St Helens WA11 9UL

ISBN 0 333 78202 X

9 8 7 6 5 4 3

A CIP catalogue record for this book is available from
the British Library.

Photography by Lesley Howling
All illustrations by Raymond Turvey (except p.34, p.36,
p.59, p.100, p.237, p.260 by Debbie Hinks, and p.31, p.83,
p.250 (left), p.259, p.261 by Cath Knox)
Designed by Macmillan General Books Design Department

Colour Reproduction by Speedscan Ltd
Printed and bound in Great Britain by Bath Press

Contents

THE BASICS

The Beginner's Programme   27

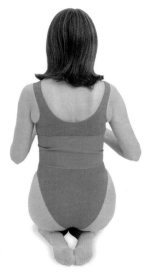

Intermediate programme   91

Advanced Programme   139

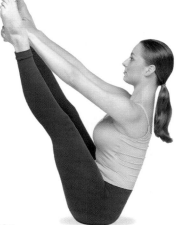

THE PRESCRIPTIONS

Body Control Pilates at Work   183

Body Control Pilates At Work At Play   199

Body Control Pilates and the Performing Arts   225

Body Control Pilates For Health   233

Glossary   265

What Next?   267

Further Information   268

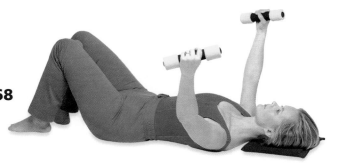

Acknowledgements

A big thank you to all the Body Control Pilates team, Jenny, Margaret and Janet who work so hard behind the scenes. A special thank you to Jenny and Margaret who are even there for me at three in the morning! I will continue to be grateful for the encouragement and confidence that Michael Alcock (my agent), Gordon Wise (Macmillan), Gareth Watson (Telstar) and David Yates (Zen Pictures) have shown in me. As for my co-authors, years of experience have finally culminated in this book, thank you for sharing your knowledge. Helge, thank you for being you! And last but by no means least, a huge thank you to my family, Leigh, Rebecca and Emily, who continue to thrive and survive despite my long absences.

Lynne Robinson

My biggest thanks you goes to my supportive husband Paul and my wonderful children Naomi and Amina. My family means a lot to me.

A special thank goes to Paul McLinden, Karen Hay and Ruth Prior for looking after our clients so well when I am away.

I am also very grateful for Leigh's friendship, support, help and hard work. We would not be here without you!

Jenny, Andrea and Margaret are a great support team in the office.

I would also like to thank all my clients, working with you inspires me and allows me to develop further.

My friends Andrea and Anja are very special to me.

Finally I would like to thank my co-authors. Especially Lynne, whose enthusiasm and energy has helped to create the copy you hold in your hands.

Helge Fisher

My thanks go to Mark Oliver, my physiotherapist in Perth, Western Australia, who initially introduced me to Pilates back in 1993.

The co-authors of this book and the Pilates teachers who have taught me so much more than a series of exercises.

Jacqueline Knox MCSP SRP

I will always be grateful to Lynne, Helge and Jackie for the continued support of our books and for making Body Control Pilates a resounding success, here and abroad. I must also thank Macmillan, especially Gordon Wise, Liz Davis and Neil Lang, who have been responsible for promoting us to a household name in the last three years. Furthermore, I should like to acknowledge the support of Cheryl, Judy, Ellena, Paul, Elle and Simone, with very special thanks to Mitsi Pippa, who has shared her knowledge and expertise with myself and all my staff. She will be sorely missed by all her colleagues, when she returns to Athens. Finally, I will always be indebted to Mum and Dad and all my loyal clients old and new.

Gordon Thomson

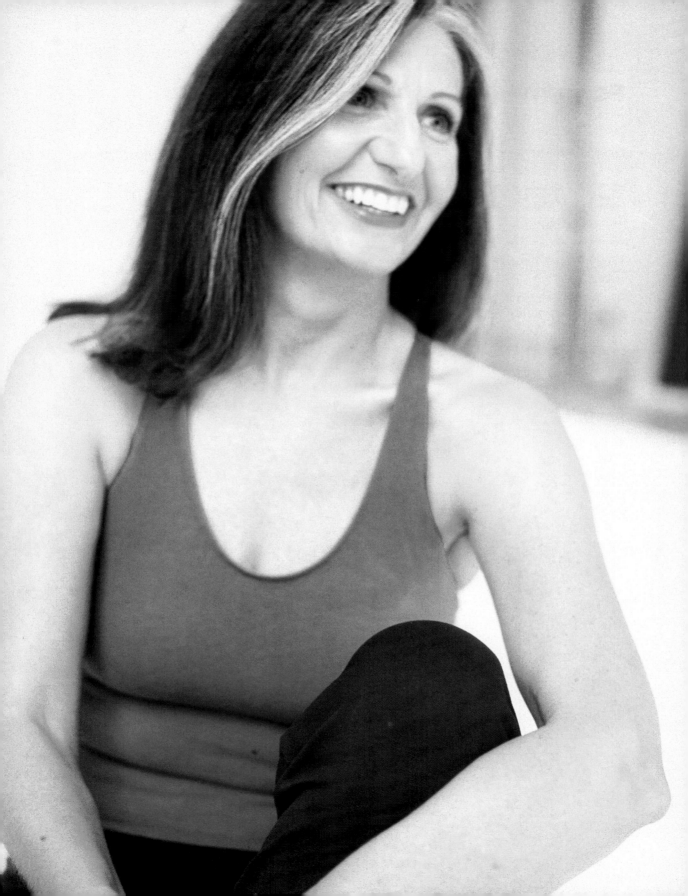

Foreword

This is *the* book that we have been eager to write and that we hope you have been waiting to read! We feel the time is right to bring all the elements of Body Control Pilates together, combining the latest medical knowledge with everything that we have learnt over the last few exciting years.

And what years they have been! Since the publication of our first book *Body Control: The Pilates Way* in 1997, we have written three further books, the last *Pilates: The Way Forward* going straight into the national bestseller listings. Meanwhile, the first book has now been translated into six languages and is sold worldwide, we have three bestselling videos – and even a 'music for Pilates' CD, *Body Control Pilates: Music for Pilates and Relaxation*! Our feet don't seem to have touched the ground in the last three years.

Why is Body Control Pilates such a phenomenal success story? How has it gone from being virtually unknown to approaching a household name? To be honest, the answer lies not in the fact that we are great literary talents, marketing geniuses or TV personalities but, rather, in the simple truth that this method of exercise works and works brilliantly, delivering all of its promises. Backed by leading physiotherapists, chiropractors and osteopaths, we have now the honour of working with élite athletes from many of England's national and Olympic teams.

But whether you are a top athlete or a first-time exerciser, a housewife or a busy executive, once you have tried exercising The Pilates Way, we know that you will get results and hope that you will feel as passionately about Body Control Pilates as we do.

Lynne Robinson

Introduction

Step by step, you can change the way you look, the way you feel and the way you move. If you want a new body – reshaped, rebalanced and realigned – a body that is longer, leaner, more supple and yet with a hidden strength, then this book is for you. It is the ultimate guide to Body Control Pilates.

This is the complete, comprehensive, easy-to-follow guide to the Body Control Pilates method of exercise, a book that will bring together much of the background information contained within our previous books and yet will take the reader further, much further. The end product, therefore, is a self-help manual which will guide you step by step through a Beginner's Programme, progressing to an Intermediate Programme and culminating in an Advanced Programme which includes the fabulous Series of Five classical Pilates exercises.

Along the way, we will give you the very latest, cutting-edge medical thinking on movement and why movement problems occur, explaining these concepts simply and relating them to the Pilates Method.

In order for you to get the most from the exercises, they should be tailored to your own personal needs. With this in mind, we have included a self-analysis section which examines the different common postural types and offers remedial programmes to help bring your body back into correct alignment.

Finally, we have studied the sort of difficulties faced by people in different occupations, sports and other sectors and offer advice on how to avoid developing injuries and problems.

Equipped with this knowledge, you will be able to work out for yourself the best possible combination of exercises so that you can achieve maximum results.

Who Is This Book For?

Everyone, because we all move and because Pilates is all about natural flowing movement. Practised regularly and correctly, Pilates will, literally, change the way you move. So, whether you are already a convert to this method – and with several hundred thousand copies of our books and videos now sold throughout the world we know there are a lot of Pilates 'fans' out there – or whether you have never before encountered this strange-sounding exercise regime, you will find this book invaluable.

When followed correctly, these exercises will change the way you look, the way you feel and the way you move! And that's a promise.

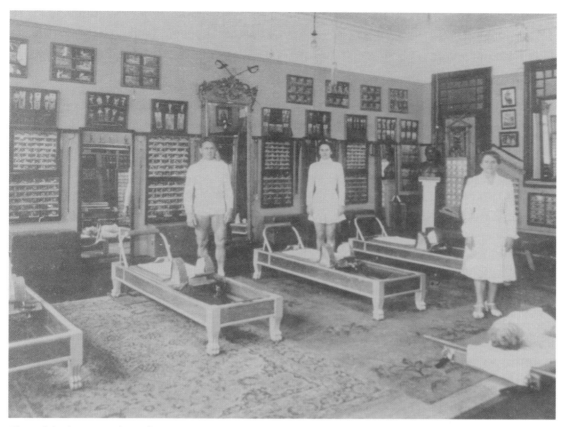

The original New York studio

Joseph Hubertus Pilates 1880–1967

When embarking on any health or fitness routine it is comforting to know that its originator lived to the ripe old age of eighty-seven! Joseph Pilates was born in Düsseldorf in 1880. He was a frail, sickly child who suffered from rickets, asthma and rheumatic fever. He was determined to overcome this fragility but instead of following an established fitness regime, he experimented with many different approaches and one can, in fact, recognize the different elements of these methods in his teaching. Yoga, gymnastics, skiing, self-defence,

dance, circus training and weight training all influenced him, and he chose aspects of each to develop his own body. By absorbing these other methods and selecting the most effective features, Pilates was able to work out a system which had the perfect balance of strength and flexibility.

Having proven their worth on his own body, he then began to teach these techniques to others. He was training detectives at Scotland Yard when the First World War broke out and because of his nationality he was interned in Lancashire and then the Isle of Man. With time on his hands, he helped out in the camp infirmary and further developed his techniques training his fellow internees with amazing success. Many of them were war veterans who had been horrendously wounded and these injuries had, in some cases, resulted in amputations. Much of his knowledge of rehabilitation comes from this period.

At the end of the war he returned to Germany where he taught self-defence to the Hamburg police and the German army. In 1926, he decided to emigrate to the United States of America. On the boat he met his future wife Clara and, when they realized they shared the same views on fitness, they decided to set up a studio in New York. This attracted top ballet dancers (many sent from George Balanchine and Martha Graham), actors and actresses, gymnasts and athletes, all anxious to learn from Pilates.

Joseph Pilates wrote several books on fitness. The exercises he describes in them are very advanced and reflect the nature of his studio clientele.

Pilates' interest was in the overall health of his clients: he advocated skin brushing long before it became generally popular and was also keen on fresh air on the body – he would often teach in his swimming trunks! One major principle dominates his work: there must be commitment to the exercises, no excuses, they must be done regularly in order to realize results.

Pilates never took the initiative of setting up an official training programme with the result that many of his disciples went on to teach their own versions of his method. The definition of what was, or is, true Pilates is therefore somewhat blurred and, indeed, is still being debated today. It is not helped by the fact that Pilates rarely taught the same exercise in the same way two days running, partly because he geared his teaching to the needs of the individual and prescribed a completely different set of exercises for each client. Some of these clients themselves went on to teach, each one therefore, working with a different emphasis.

The Development of Body Control Pilates

The Pilates Method has now been taught for some eighty years, but it is only recently that the medical profession has really begun to look closely at why the system is so successful. Before this, many Pilates teachers taught intuitively, learning through apprenticeship about good alignment and good body use but, in many cases, without fully knowing the technical medical terms for what they were doing. Under the close scrutiny of the medical world, we have had to re-examine our methods and study precisely why they work so well.

This has been a great advantage to Pilates teachers as they have been able to absorb new ideas in physiotherapy techniques and movement therapies, for example, and incorporate them into the Method without sacrificing its uniqueness. As a result, Pilates continues to evolve without the constraint of a rigid set of rules.

The Body Control Pilates Method has developed from the work of Joseph Pilates, and been refined by Lynne Robinson, Gordon Thomson and Helge Fisher. Body Control Pilates is unique in the way that it prepares the body for the classical Pilates exercises. Few people today could start their first session

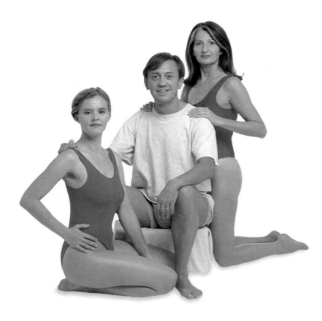

ciently large, the intention of the founders was to develop more specialized activities to meet the growing need for Pilates-type applications in sport and medicine. During those early days, we had no idea that the response would be such that, within three years, those activities would already be fully established and up and running!

The first book *Body Control: The Pilates Way* quickly became an international bestseller and played a key role in fuelling the worldwide surge in Pilates that has occurred in the last two years or so. This has meant that one of our key tasks now is, in fact, to control this growth in such a way that we can continue to guarantee the quality and maintain the strong reputation of the Body Control Pilates Method. In recent months, as the number of companies offering short Pilates teacher-training courses has grown considerably, we have chosen to raise the standards for qualification as a Body Control Pilates teacher to maintain our position as a quality standard.

The Body Control Pilates group is now based in Covent Garden, London, from where its various businesses are steered. The Body Control Pilates Teacher Training organization has gone from strength to strength and, as well as introducing more specialized courses for existing teachers, has now started working internationally with the establishment of centres in Belgium and Austria. The Body Control Pilates Institute was launched in September 1999 with the aim of offering specialist training and programmes for the sectors of sport and medicine. Apart from the regular workshops and courses run in hospitals, the Institute has already started working closely with the English Football Association, the English Cricket Board, several professional football clubs and leading individuals from a variety of sports. Among its other activities, the group also operates several Body Control Pilates studios and, notable in this, is the

with the Full Hundred (page 148) as was traditionally the case. We believe that you need to acquire the skills to perform such exercises gradually and this progressive approach has won the respect and support of leading medical bodies as well as top sports associations.

This has led to an explosive expansion in the total Body Control Pilates activity since it was 'launched' in 1996 from a small office above Gordon's South Kensington studio. Three main goals existed at that time: first, to develop and implement a programme for training new teachers in the Body Control Pilates method; second, to set up a legally-constituted professional Pilates body which could liaise with government and industry as well as support the intended international network of qualified teachers; third, to begin the task of building a wider pubic awareness of the Method and the benefits it offers.

Once the base was built and, most importantly, the number of qualified teachers became suffi-

close working relationship developed with the David Lloyd Leisure network of health and racquet clubs whereby the Body Control Pilates group runs classes in all the clubs as well as operating a number of fully equipped studios.

The international growth in interest has also meant that, over the last two years or so, Lynne, Gordon and Helge have accepted invitations to visit countries as varied as South Africa, Thailand, Tunisia, Germany, Austria, Jamaica and Belgium to lecture or run workshops and courses.

Alongside the training and commercial activities, The Body Control Pilates Association has now become the largest professional Pilates organization outside the United States of America. It is a non-profit making body whose members work to a Code of Practice regarding teaching standards and professional ethics. Only those teachers who are suitably qualified and who work to this Code are able to use the Body Control Pilates 'label' for their classes. Sadly, as Pilates has become more popular, many of the new classes starting up round the country are run by teachers who either have minimal formal training, or often none whatsoever, in the Pilates Methods. The responsible players in the Pilates industry have responded to this by working together to define a standard that all teachers should meet before they can properly call themselves Pilates teachers. However, one golden rule remains before you join any Pilates class – or any other fitness class – ask the teacher whether they hold a recognized qualification and how long their training programme was. A good course will have a structured curriculum taught in modules, a practical assessment, a written examination and a period of supervised teaching. This takes three months, not days.

We often say that Pilates is a continuous learning process and almost every presentation or workshop that we run throws up new ideas or information which we do our best to take on board and bring into our training or teaching where appropriate. So it is also with the various Body Control Pilates books and videos that have been released (see the back of this book for more details). We do our best to incorporate into each new book the latest developments with regard to exercise and technique and the latest medical research – in this respect, we are very fortunate to work closely with a team of leading physiotherapists and sports scientists who act as advisors to the Body Control Pilates group.

This manual represents, therefore, the summation of our combined experience and of our own continued learning process. It is intended to become *the* reference book for The Body Control Pilates Method, including not only the latest research but explaining how Body Control Pilates can be applied to everyday life, whether at work or at play.

The Benefits of the Pilates Method

- Improved flexibility
- Greater strength and muscle tone
- More efficient respiratory system
- More efficient lymphatic system therefore less toxins in the body
- More efficient circulatory system
- Lowered stress levels
- A flatter stomach and a trimmer waist through the creation of a natural girdle of strength
- Better posture

- Toned buttocks and thighs
- Toned arms and shoulder area
- Fewer headaches (where they are posture-based)
- Less incidence of back pain
- Boosted immune system
- Increased bone density
- Greater joint mobility
- Fewer injuries for dancers/athletes
- Improved performance for dancers/athletes

How To Use This Book

The idea of this book is to take you step by step through the Body Control Pilates programme, slowly increasing your strength, your flexibility and your body awareness. We will give you all the information you need to 'customize' your sessions, tailoring them to your individual needs, so that you get maximum results. Before you begin the exercises, study the different postural types on pages 13–16 and try to determine which type you most closely resemble. If you find this difficult, your practitioner (physiotherapist, chiropractor or osteopath) should be able to advise you. Make a note of the exercises recommended for your postural type, then look to see if any of the special sections later in the book are relevant to you. If they are, again make a note of the exercises we recommend. These can then be combined with those for your postural type.

Armed with this information, you can start the Beginner's Programme, gradually working your way through the programme but taking special note of your 'recommended' exercises which should be included each time you practise. It may be that we

have recommended an exercise from the level above the one you are at. Leave this out until you are ready. Only move on to the next level, intermediate, when you are completely familiar, and comfortable, with the Beginner's Programme. Do not be too ambitious. It takes many months on average to reach intermediate level and many more again to achieve advanced level. We cannot give you a set time frame as no two people are the same: it depends on your overall fitness, age, physical history, injuries and more. However, please bear in mind that for the lay person it can take several years before you gain the necessary skills and strength to perform the Series of Five!

Try to do about three hours' exercise a week. This can be divided in several ways, thirty minutes a day, three one-hour sessions or two ninety-minute sessions. Generally speaking, thirty minutes a day is the best way to start as it will remind your body how it should be moving. As you progress to the intermediate and advanced levels, the longer sessions become more valuable.

Natural Flowing Movement

First we need to consider how movement takes place and then we can examine what may go wrong and why.

Imagine for a moment that you are standing watching normal healthy children play. How do they move? Easily, freely, without inhibition or restriction, with natural flowing movements. Their bodies have it all: grace, strength, stamina, suppleness, speed. You don't see children stretching before they jump on the climbing frame; they don't need to – they don't have tight muscles – they have bodies which work, and work well, because they are constantly on the move. If you liken the whole range of movements which we are capable of performing to the alphabet, then children use every single letter, 'A–Z', construct sentences and write stories. Now, imagine a similar group of adults. How many letters of the alphabet do adults use? We rarely get past 'E'. As adults we continually repeat the same movements day in, day out. What you put into the body, you get out. If you don't use it, you'll lose the ability. Why?

There are three parts to your body's movement:

- The nervous system – telephone, control
- The skeletal structure – passive: bones, joints, ligaments, cartilage,
- The musculature – active

A good example of this is if you were to stand on one leg – let's say your right leg – for twenty minutes, your brain would 'forget' your left leg existed. When you tried to put your weight on it again, it would feel numb. The brain continually tells the body to react and adapt to stimuli or lack of stimuli.

Movement depends on messages to and from the control room of the brain; there is a constant flow of input and output. What is starting to come to the fore in medical research is the importance of good input. The brain remembers patterns of movement, not individual muscle contractions. By repeating sound movement patterns and by moving correctly, you change the input. This has an amazing effect on how you move. If the brain receives the right messages these will be locked into the muscle memory banks.

By restricting your movements or by moving incorrectly, you can invite problems.

'It is the mind itself which builds the body'
Joseph Pilates' favourite quote, from Schiller

Back now to our children playing . . . what happens to the free movement as they grow, where does it go? Up to the age of five, the freedom is still there and then we sit them down at school for hours on end on tiny chairs in front of desks where they fidget and get discouraged; we pile on the homework and exams, so their stress levels rise; they carry heavily loaded backpacks over one shoulder distorting the spine and musculature. When they reach puberty, their bodies often become an imagined source of embarrassment, slouching becomes cool.

Later on in the workplace, the chances are that they will sit at a desk, at a till or behind a steering wheel all day and then drive home to sit on the couch all evening. Where's the movement now, the stimulation, the input? It is restricted to a few repetitive actions. Muscle is dependent upon, and reflects, patterns of use. Disuse and/or misuse is associated with changes in muscle function. By not using your muscles properly, you particularly affect the anti-gravity postural muscles that lie deep within the body. It is these muscles which support (or stabilize) the spine and other joints. If they weaken, other muscles will take on their role and muscle imbalances then occur.

So how do we undo the damage, how do we reverse years of bad body use?

We start from scratch. Slowly re-learning and re-educating the body in how to move correctly again. The nervous system is incredibly flexible and adaptable and will reorganize itself as a result of training. There are three stages to this process, each stage leading to the next:

- Thinking about good movement (awareness)
- Practising good movement
- The movements will then become 'automatic' or 'grooved', the muscle remembers them. This is known as muscle memory engram

This is where Pilates is perfect. The programme we recommend will take you progressively through the stages needed to change your existing movement patterns, ensuring that every action is performed correctly which will restore natural, normal movement.

Strength from Within

Back to muscles, the active part of the equation. Muscles work together in groups to move our bones. They work as a team. While one muscle may act as the main mover (agonist), the opposing muscles have to pay out to allow the movement to take place (antagonist), and others are involved to fix the bones in the right place (stabilizers) or to add subtle variation (synergists). With everything working correctly and firing up in the right order or sequence you have a good pattern of use, a sound recruitment pattern and normal movement. That's exactly how we used to move as children but over

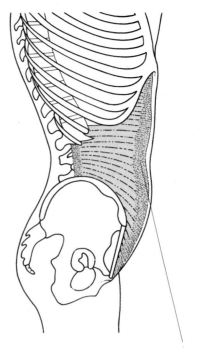

*Transversus Abdominus
(your girdle of strength)*

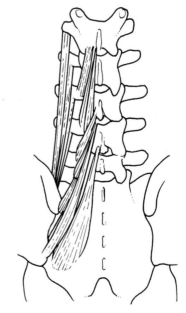

Multifidus

Muscle Fibres

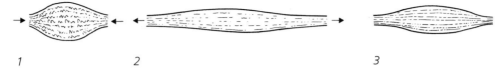

1   2   3

1. If a muscle is shorter than its ideal length it cannot function effectively
2. Longer than ideal length and it cannot function effectively
3. Muscles must be the right length and have the right type of fibres to work effectively

time, all sorts of factors contribute to a loss of normal movement and to postural misalignments. This is going to affect every movement we make.

The importance of the stabilizing muscles is becoming increasingly clear in medical research. Let's say for a moment that you want to reach up to take a book from a high shelf. Which muscles do you think would be the first to engage? The hand or shoulder muscles perhaps? The answer is the deep postural muscles, those which support the spine. It makes sense. You don't want to fall over while you reach up. These deep muscles – the transversus abdominis, the pelvic floor and a deep back muscle called multifidus – are the ones which stabilize the lumbar spine, ensuring that one vertebra doesn't shear too far off its neighbour.

These muscles engage to form a natural corset, a 'girdle of strength', round your centre so that the movement can take place easily and smoothly and safely. You must have this stable base, in the same way that a tower crane needs a stable base while the long arm moves round.

Problems can arise when these deep stabilizing muscles are not working correctly. This was the subject of 'Muscle Control – Pain Control: What Exercises Would You Prescribe?' an article by G. A. Jull and C. A. Richardson published in 1995 in *Manual Therapy*. This can happen when the body is out of its correct alignment and held in incorrect positions for sustained periods of time. The stabilizing muscles are held on a stretch, they weaken and other muscles are forced to take over the stabilizing role. You then have the situation of the wrong muscles doing the wrong job and the birth of a faulty recruitment pattern, a pattern of misuse. In order for a muscle to work efficiently, it needs to be at its optimum length. When it is held overstretched or overlengthened it cannot work effectively, neither will it work properly if it is held overshortened.

Simply speaking, you can think of muscles as having two types of role: a stabilizing role, that is holding bones in place; or a mobilizing role, that is creating large movements. In an ideal world muscles destined to stabilize will stabilize, those designed to mobilize will mobilize. Returning to our image of the crane, the stabilizers are the stable base, the

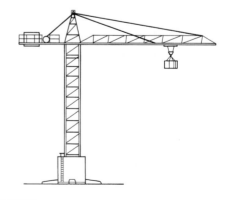

The crane

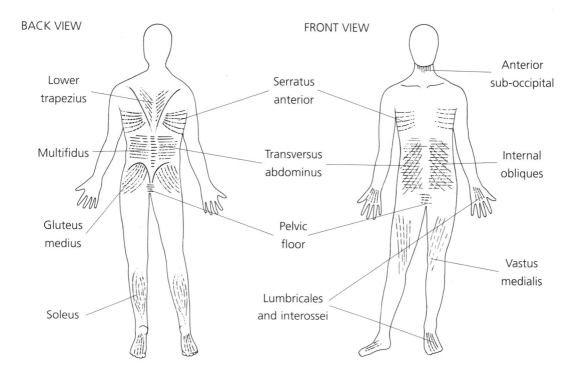

BACK VIEW

FRONT VIEW

Lower trapezius

Multifidus

Gluteus medius

Soleus

Serratus anterior

Transversus abdominus

Pelvic floor

Lumbricales and interossei

Anterior sub-occipital

Internal obliques

Vastus medialis

The main stabilizers targeted by Pilates exercises

mobilizers make the large sweeping movements of the arm of the crane.

These two types of muscles have different characteristics. Stabilizing muscles have to work for long periods of time, they have to hold tone and need endurance. They usually lie deeper within the body and are often shorter in length than mobilizing muscles. They work at about 20–30 per cent of their full efficiency or Maximum Voluntary Contraction (MVC).

Mobilizing muscles, on the other hand, make big movements, such as moving the limbs round. In order to do this they work in phases, turning on and off. They tend to lie closer to the surface than stabilizing muscles and are usually quite long, they fatigue quickly and work at between 40–100 per cent of their full efficiency (MVC).

Some muscles need to work as stabilizers in some movements and mobilizers in others. If, however, a deep stabilizing muscle is not functioning properly due to weakness, a mobilizer may take on a stabilizing role. As an example, your hamstring muscles, at the back of your thighs, which for many movements act as mobilizing muscles making larger movements, are often 'obliged' to take on the role of stabilizing the pelvis because the deep gluteals (buttocks) are too weak. Consequently they tighten and shorten. No amount of stretching will lengthen them while they have to keep stabilizing. The solution to this problem would be to strengthen the deep gluteals and enable the hamstrings to let go!

When these two types of muscles, stabilizers and mobilizers, work perfectly at their own jobs, the

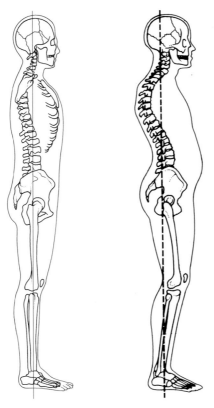

Ideal plumbline alignment.
Figure one

Kyphosis-Lordosis.
Figure two

body is balanced, all the groups of muscles work in synergy and joints are held in their most favourable position, which is their natural 'neutral' position. You can see this in a person with perfect posture.

By studying figure one, you can see that all the joints in the body are held in their optimum natural position. When this person moves, with good muscle recruitment and with the stabilizing muscles working correctly, there is going to be minimal wear and tear on his joints. Good input

is received by the brain and is locked into the memory banks.

Compare this with figure two. Here, most of the joints are held out of their natural, neutral positions because of existing muscle imbalances. Tight, short-ened muscles and weak, lengthened muscles, inefficient stabilizers and overactive mobilizers equal faulty recruitment patterns which feel like normal movement. As these patterns of misuse are repeated the input to the nervous system accepts them as normal, the brain received bad input which it locks into its memory bank.

So, in order to change the way we move we have to go back to basics and change the input, rebalancing the role of stabilizing and mobilizing muscles so we get the right muscles doing the right jobs. Then, by repeating these good movement patterns, the brain will receive the correct input and natural, normal movement will be restored to the body.

All the exercises in this book are designed to do just this. The detailed directions which you are given about the position of your pelvis and shoulders, about your breathing and about engaging your abdominal muscles make us unlike any other fitness technique. It means that you will have to be patient and build your strength gradually. There are no shortcuts. We have to develop your proprioceptive skills, your kinaesthetic sense, that is, your aware-ness of where you are in space – of what exactly your limbs are doing – which is based on the constant two-way communication channels. This body awareness lies at the heart of the matter. When you know what you are doing as you move, you will automatically engage the right muscles and the rest will follow.

Recognizing your Postural Type

Many of the problems seen by physiotherapists, chiropractors and osteopaths are related to poor posture. We now need to look at what we mean by 'poor'. To do this, let's look first at 'ideal posture'.

With ideal posture the forces of gravity are evenly distributed through the body, so all joints are in their neutral zone. There will be minimal wear and tear on these structures and the natural balance and correct length of the muscles is maintained. Muscles are balanced, therefore movement patterns are normal. All vital organs are properly placed and not constricted, so they function better.

Notice the points of the body through which the imaginary plumb line falls:

- The ear lobe
- The bodies of the cervical vertebrae (the neck)
- The tip of the shoulder
- Dividing the thorax (ribcage) in half
- The bodies of the lumbar vertebrae
- Slightly behind the hip joint
- Slightly in front of the centre of the knee joint
- Slightly in front of the lateral malleolus (outside ankle bone)

This, then, is what we should all aspire to, bearing in mind that we each have our own distinctive body shape, size and dimensions.

So what goes wrong? We can summarize the factors which may influence your posture:

- Hereditary factors (if your mother was kyphotic – see above – for example, there is every chance that you will be too)
- Injuries
- Illness, mental and physical
- Work-related factors, the type of job you do
- Hobby/sport related influences can create muscle imbalances

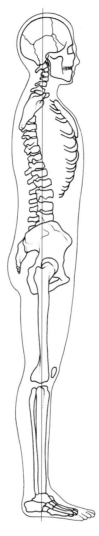

The head is in neutral neither tilted forward or back

The shoulder blades (scapulae) lie flat against the thorax

The ribcage is not compressed so breathing is more efficient

The spine retains its natural curves

The pelvis is in neutral (the anterior superior iliac spine in a parallel line with the pubis symphysis)

The knee joints are in a line and not hyper-extended (locked back)

The lower leg is vertical and at a right angle to the sole of the foot

Ideal plumbline alignment

- Environmental influences
- Emotional issues
- Sustained positions
- Repetitive movements
- Fashion and culture

(It is interesting to note that left- or right-handedness may result in altered patterns of movement and skeletal alignment, but these are not considered faulty postures.)

All these factors may have an effect on our bodies and may change us from having the ideal posture seen above to one of the three types below.

Identifying the postural type which you fit is not always easy. Sometimes, we are combinations of those shown below. The best way to be sure is to stand in your underwear, side on to a mirror, and get someone to hold a plumb line (a piece of string with a weight attached) and then compare this to the diagrams above, noticing where the plumb line falls in relation to each postural type. But if you are in any doubt, consult your Pilates teacher or your practitioner for advice.

Posture Type One: Kyphosis-Lordosis

This first posture type is very common. What has happened? Notice where the plumb line falls now:

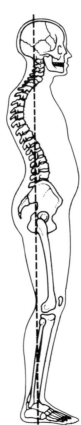

Kyphosis-Lordosis

- The head is thrust forward shortening the back of the neck, the chin juts forward so that the neck flexors are weak and the neck extensors short and strong.

- The upper back: the thoracic spine is overly-rounded. A kyphosis just means a curvature but in this case it would be more appropriate to talk about there being too much of a kyphosis. As a result, the muscles at the front of the chest (anterior deltoids) and pectorals are tight and shortened, those at the back of the thorax are held lengthened and are therefore weak (especially lower trapezius). The shoulder blades are most probably abducted, that is they have moved outwards away from the ribcage. The thoracic back extensors are lengthened. This is also known as Upper Crossed Syndrome.

- The pelvis is, anteriorly rotated – tilted forward. Any change in the position of the pelvis will have an effect on the spine and the hips. In this case the spine has too much of a curve, it is overly hollowed, hyperextended.

- The muscles of the low back, the superficial erector spinae, are shortened.

- The hip flexors are shortened.

- The abdominals are inevitably very weak.

- The hamstrings are usually tight because they are substituting for weak gluteals.

- Weak gluteals.

- The knees are slightly hyperextended.

The exercises we recommend for this postural type are as follows:

Relaxation Position	p.28	
The Compass	p.31	
Pelvic Stability	p.38	
Shoulder Drops	p.48	

Neck Rolls	p.50	
Spine Curls	p.45	
Hip Flexor Stretch (Side-Lying Quadriceps Stretch also good)	p.47 (p.84)	
Side Rolls	p.54	
Hamstring Stretch	p.82	
Curl Ups	p.78	
Oblique Curl Ups	p.79	
The Arm Weights Series: Flys (but without weights)	p.125	
The Dart or The Diamond Press	p.70 or p.110	
The Star	p.114	
Rest Position	p.73	
Sliding Down the Wall	p.66	
The Corkscrew	p.96	
The Dumb Waiter	p.56	
Pole Raises	p.60	
Arm Openings	p.52	
Chalk Circle	p.136	

Posture Type Two: The Swayback

This posture is often seen combined with the last and is particularly popular among teenagers who have mastered the art of slouching!

- The head is forward of the plumb line, so once again the neck flexors are weak.
- The thoracic spine has swayed noticeably backwards.
- The upper abdominals may be short, the lower weak.
- The thoracic back extensors are lengthened.
- The pelvis is tilted back-wards but moved slightly forward of the plumb line, resulting in the pelvis swaying forward in relation to the feet.
- The curvature of the lumbar spine is reduced and flattened.
- The hip flexors are long and weak.
- The hamstrings are short and strong.
- The band of muscle that runs down the side of the legs, the tensor fasciae latae, can be short.
- The gluteals are often noticeably weak and wobbly!
- The hip joints are in extension, as are the knees which are often held locked back.

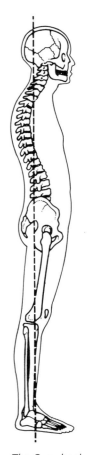

The Swayback

The exercises we recommend for this postural type are as follows:

Spine Curls	p.45	
Pelvic Stability, especially Knee Folds	p.39	
Curl Ups	p.78	
Oblique Curl Ups	p.79	
Single Leg Stretch (when ready)	p.106	
Hamstring Stretch	p.82	
Side Reach	p.64	
Table Top	p.81	
The Diamond Press	p.110	
The Dart	p.70	
The Star	p.114	
The Big Squeeze	p.72	
Rest Position	p.73	
Arm Openings or Chalk Circle	p.52 or p.136	

Posture Type Three: The Flatback

This is relatively easy to spot as the back is flat!

- The head is again forward of the plumb line so the neck flexors will be weak.
- The thoracic area is interesting as the upper section can be rounded while the lower part is quite straight.
- The pelvis is obviously tilted backwards.
- The hamstrings are short and tight (which pulls the back of the pelvis down).
- The hip flexors on the other hand are long and weak.
- The upper abdominals are often short.
- Usually the knee joints are hyper-extended but occasionally they can be held flexed.

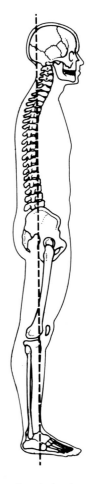

The Flatback

The exercises we recommend for this postural type are as follows:

Roll Downs	p.68	
Spine Curls	p.45	
Side Rolls	p.54	
Hamstring Stretches	p.82	
Curl Ups	p.78	
Oblique Curl Ups	p.79	
Threading a Needle	p.77	
Beach Ball Hamstring Stretch	p.123	
The Star	p.114	
The Big Squeeze	p.72	
Rest Position	p.73	
The Cossack	p.31	
Pole Raises	p.60	
Arm Openings or Chalk Circle	p.52 or p.136	

Combining Exercises for Your Postural Type

To give you an example of how to combine exercises, let's say that you are a cricketer with a swayback posture. A typical one hour workout for you would be:

Four Point kneeling	p.35	
Relaxation Position	p.28	
The Starfish	p.42	
Pelvic Stability	p.38	
Spine Curls	p.45	
Curl Ups	p.78	
Oblique Curl Ups	p.79	
Hamstring Stretch	p.82	
Side Rolls, when stable	p.54	
Pole Raises	p.60	
The Corkscrew	p.96	
The Dart	p.70	
The Star	p.114	
The Big Squeeze	p.72	

Rest Position	p.73	
Table Top, sliding legs	p.119	
Rest Position	p.73	
Arm Openings/Chalk Circle	p.52 or p.136	

With a swayback posture your hip flexors are usually lengthened therefore you would leave out the hip flexor stretch.

Another example: a sedentary worker with a Kyphosis-Lordosis posture:

The Starfish	p.42	
Pelvic Stability	p.38	
Shoulder Drops	p.48	
Neck Rolls	p.50	
Spine Curls	p.45	
Hip Flexor Stretch	p.47	

Side Rolls	p.54	
Hamstring Stretch	p.82	
Curl Ups	p.78	
Oblique Curl Ups	p.79	
Side-lying Quadriceps Stretch	p.84	
Flys without weights	p.125	
The Dart or The Diamond Press	p.70 or p.110	
The Star	p.114	
Rest Position	p.73	
The Corkscrew	p.96	
The Cossack	p.62	
The Dumb Waiter	p.56	
Pole Raises	p.60	
Arm Openings	p.52	

The Eight Principles of Pilates

- Relaxation
- Concentration
- Alignment
- Breathing
- Centring
- Co-ordination
- Flowing Movements
- Stamina

Relaxation

This is the starting point for everyone when they begin to learn Pilates. It may seem a strange way to begin an exercise routine, most of you being more accustomed to jogging on the spot or stretching but our first priority is to ensure that you bring none of the stress of the day into your session. Learning how to recognize and release areas of unwanted tension is a must before you work out, otherwise the wrong muscles will be firing up again and again and you'll never break the cycle of bad body use.

So where do most of us hold tension? The most common areas that tighten up are round the back of the neck and upper shoulders (where you always want to be massaged). But if you sit a lot, you may also find the muscles round the front of the hips can get very tight. These hip flexor muscles can also shorten when there are faulty recruitment patterns.

Our first goal in Pilates, therefore, is to teach you to be aware of tension and then how to release it. The Relaxation Position on page 28 is a good way to start your session, allowing the stress of the day to melt away into the floor. You will also notice that we use this position as the starting position for many of the exercises. As you advance in Pilates, however, you should be able to use a simple basic exercise to the same effect.

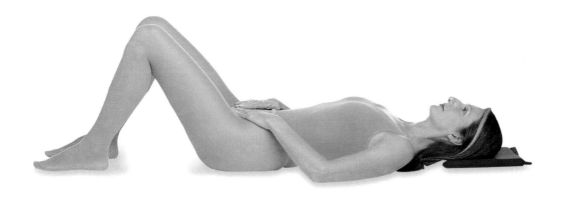

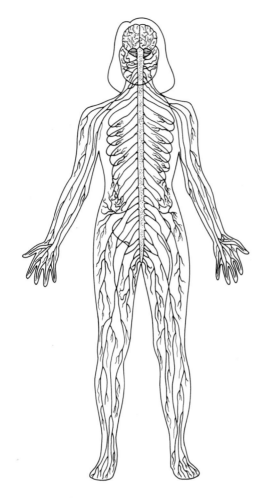

Pathways of the nervous system

Concentration

Remember: 'It is the mind itself which builds the body'. Hopefully you are now relaxed yet ready to begin to exercise. Another benefit that comes with the relaxation is that it helps you to focus. Pilates is a mental and physical conditioning programme which aims to train both the mind and the body. We have already seen how movement takes place, the importance of the constant input and output, neurological pathways and the two way communication channel.

Just like a telephone line, if there is no activity for a long period the chances are you'll get cut off!! Pilates requires you to be constantly aware of how you are moving, it requires you to focus your mind on each and every movement that you make. It develops your body's sensory feedback or kinaesthetic sense, so that you know where you are in space and what you are doing with every part of your body. Although the movements themselves may become automatic with time, you still have to concentrate, because there is always a further level of awareness to reach.

Alignment

So now you are relaxed and focused. Our next step is to bring the body into good postural alignment. By reminding it constantly of how it should be standing, sitting or lying and by moving correctly you can start to bring the body gradually back into better alignment. This, as we have seen, is essential if we are going to restore proper muscle balance. If you exercise without due attention to the correct position of the joints, you risk stressing the joint and building imbalances into the surrounding muscles. The remedial programmes given for each postural type will also help gradually to bring the body into good alignment.

Good alignment of each and every part of the body while exercising is crucial to safety and to correcting muscle imbalances. You must have your bones in the right place to get the right muscles working, in that way you build the muscles so that they will support the joint not stress it.

The following checklist should help you align your body correctly:

Allow your head to go
forward and up

Allow your neck
to release

Keep your shoulder blades
down into your back

Keep your
breastbone soft

Lengthen up through
the spine

Elbows open

Check your pelvis – is it
in neutral? (see page 31)

When you bend your knees
they should bend directly
over the centre of your foot

What about your feet
and legs? Usually, they
should be hip-width
apart and in parallel

Keep the weight
even on both feet –
do not allow them
to roll in or out

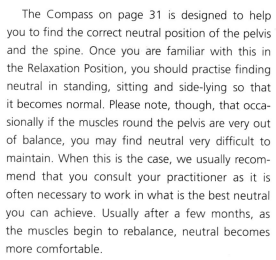

The Compass on page 31 is designed to help you to find the correct neutral position of the pelvis and the spine. Once you are familiar with this in the Relaxation Position, you should practise finding neutral in standing, sitting and side-lying so that it becomes normal. Please note, though, that occasionally if the muscles round the pelvis are very out of balance, you may find neutral very difficult to maintain. When this is the case, we usually recommend that you consult your practitioner as it is often necessary to work in what is the best neutral you can achieve. Usually after a few months, as the muscles begin to rebalance, neutral becomes more comfortable.

Nearly all our exercises should be performed in this neutral position unless you are told otherwise. You would not start your car if the gears were not in neutral, so please do not start an exercise!

Breathing

Hopefully you are now relaxed, focused and aligned, so we wish to concentrate next on improving the efficiency of your breathing.

Stand in front of a mirror and watch the way you breathe. Take a deep breath. Notice what happens to your shoulders – do they rise up round the ears accompanied by heaving bosoms (ladies only, of course)? Or perhaps your lower stomach expands when you breathe in? All these are inefficient ways of taking a breath.

So how do we want you to breathe? Wide and full into your back and sides. This makes sound sense as our lungs are situated in the ribcage and by expanding the ribcage, the volume of the cavity is increased and the capacity for oxygen intake is therefore also increased. It encourages us to make maximum use of the lower part of our lungs. This type of breathing works the muscles between the

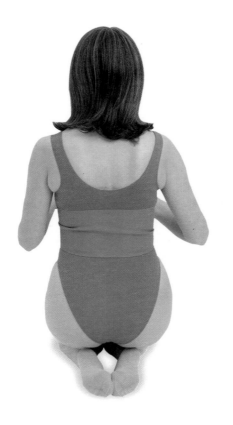

fitness regimes, but once you have mastered it, it makes sense. As a general rule, we:

Breathe in to prepare for a movement
Breathe out, strong centre to spine, and move
Breathe in to recover

Moving on the exhalation enables you to relax into the stretch and prevents you from tensing. It also offers you greater core stability at the hardest part of the exercise and safeguards against you holding your breath which can unduly stress the heart and lead to serious complications.

Centring: Creating a 'Girdle Of Strength'

It is fascinating to think that over eighty years ago Joseph Pilates discovered that if he hollowed his navel back towards his spine, his low back felt protected. He had no knowledge of the concept of 'core stability' or the transversus abdominis muscle but he had superb body awareness and thus introduced the direction 'navel to spine' into all Pilates exercises.

ribs, facilitating their expansion and making the upper body more fluid and mobile. We call it thoracic or lateral breathing. Your lungs become like bellows, the lower ribcage expanding wide as you breathe in and closing down as you breathe out. We do not wish to block the descent of the diaphragm but, rather, we encourage the movement to be widthways and into the back.

The exercise on page 29 will help you to breathe laterally.

This type of breathing is important to our way of exercising, as is the timing of the breath. You can help or hinder a movement by breathing in or out. All Pilates exercises are carefully designed to rein-force and encourage the correct muscle recruitment by using the breath. Most people find this timing difficult at first, especially if you are used to other

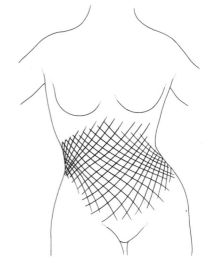

Girdle of Strength

We have moved on since then. The latest medical research indicates that the best stability is to be had if the action begins with the pelvic floor and then the lower abdominals are engaged. This is why we now use the direction 'zip up and hollow'. As you breathe out, draw up the muscles of the pelvic floor and hollow the lower abdominals back to the spine as if you are doing up this internal zip!

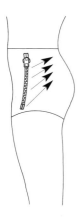

'Zip up and hollow' drawing up and in the muscles of the pelvic floor and hollowing the lower abdomen back towards the spine

You will notice that we have chosen to use the word 'hollow' to describe the action. It is very important that you do not grip your abdominals tightly for this will only create unnecessary tension and you will probably engage the wrong muscles to boot. Remember, stabilizing muscles need to be worked at 30 per cent of their full effort (MVC).

Once you have learned to create a strong centre, you can then add movements such as extension, rotation (twisting), flexion (bending forwards).

Co-ordination

You have mastered lateral breathing, correct alignment and the creation of a strong centre. Now we need to learn how to add movement to the equation while maintaining this strong centre. This isn't easy to begin with but, like learning to drive a car, it soon becomes an automatic movement – a muscle memory. Meanwhile, the actual process of learning this co-ordination is excellent mental and physical training, stimulating that two-way communication channel. Remember that the brain remembers sequences of movements so we need to feed it good movement input and sound recruitment patterns. We usually start with small movements and then build up to more complicated combinations. The idea is to challenge you constantly, to keep moving the goal posts. We may add resistance and load. Whatever exercise you are performing, however, the movements must be correctly executed, the right muscles doing the work, the right alignment, the right breathing. By the repetition of these sound movement patterns, we can start to change the way you move!

Flowing Movements

Pilates is all about natural movements performed correctly, gracefully and with control. You will not be required to twist into any awkward positions or to strain. Movements are generally slow, lengthening away from the strong centre. This gives you the opportunity to check your alignment and to focus on using the right muscles to do the job. You can also stop if you feel any discomfort, making Pilates one of the safest forms of exercise. Slow doesn't mean easy though – in fact it is harder to do an exercise slowly than quickly, and it is also less easy to cheat!

Stamina

Finally, we aim to build endurance into our key muscles. This is achieved as you progressively challenge your stability. As you become more proficient at the exercises and your muscles begin to work the way nature intended, you will discover that your overall stamina will improve dramatically. You will no longer be wasting energy holding on to unnecessary tension or moving inefficiently. Many people complain of tiredness after a day on their feet, simply because standing badly is tiring. The ribcage is compressed and, as a consequence, the lungs are constricted. As you learn to open and lengthen the body, breathing becomes more efficient. All Pilates exercises are designed to encourage the respiratory, lymphatic and circulatory systems to function more effectively. Think of a well-serviced car where the engine is tuned and the wheels aligned – it runs more efficiently as will your body!

The only thing that Pilates doesn't offer is cardio-vascular work. Having said that, The Series of Five on page 174, when performed in succession, will increase the heart rate but, generally speaking, you will need to add some aerobic work into your fitness programme. Brisk walking, cycling, swimming (backstroke especially) are all excellent but please bear in mind that you must use your body well while doing them or you will undo all the good you have done in your Pilates session.

What Pilates can do is make you fit for your chosen sport or activity. It will ensure that you use your body correctly with sound movement patterns while you run, play tennis or swim. It will help to prepare the body before your activity and rebalance it afterwards.

The Eight Principles Summarized

Relaxation
Take a few minutes at the start of each session to release unwanted tension from the body. Ideally this should be done in the Relaxation Position (page 28). Alternatively, you may use exercises such as Beach Ball Hamstrings or Roll Downs (advanced exercises) to prepare the body and the mind.

Concentration
Clear your mind, and focus on your body as you exercise. Concentrate on each and every movement so that you are 'in' the movement itself, totally aware.

Alignment
Use this concentration to ensure that you are correctly placed before you exercise and while you move.

Breathing
Use lateral breathing. Breathe in wide and full into your sides and your back. As you breathe out, allow your ribs to close down and your breastbone to soften. Timing: breathe in wide and full and lengthen up through the spine; breathe out, zip up and hollow and move; breathe in as you recover, staying zipped up and hollowed.

Centring
As you breathe out, zip up from the pelvic floor and hollow the lower abdominals back to the spine. Maintain the strong centre, as you move and as you breathe in. You must create a strong centre before you move.

Co-ordination

Co-ordinate your alignment, your breathing, your centring with your movements. Start with simple movements such as The Starfish (page 42) and build up to the more advanced complex sequences such as the Advanced Double Leg Stretch (page 154), culminating in The Series of Five!

Flowing Movements

Control all your movements, lengthening away from a strong centre. Move without strain or stress, keeping the rhythm of the particular exercise.

Stamina

Challenge your stability to improve endurance, building up your stamina slowly. Do not attempt the difficult exercises too soon. We have indicated the level of each exercise. Remember to include some aerobic work such as brisk walking as part of your weekly routine.

Before You Begin

- Be sure that you have no pressing unfinished business.
- Take the telephone off the hook, or put the answering machine on.
- You may prefer silence, otherwise put on some unobtrusive classical or ambient music.
- All exercises should be done on a padded mat.
- Wear something warm and comfortable which allows free movement.
- Barefoot is best, socks otherwise.
- The best time to exercise is in the late afternoon or evening when your muscles are already warmed up as a result of the day's activity. Exercising in the morning is fine, but you will need to take longer to warm up thoroughly.
- You will need space to work in – you cannot keep stopping to move furniture. Some clear wall space will be needed if you are going to do exercises against the wall.
- Items you may need include a chair, a small flat but firm pillow for behind your head or perhaps a folded towel, a larger pillow, a long scarf and a tennis ball.

Please do not exercise if:

- You are feeling unwell.
- You have just eaten a heavy meal.
- You have been drinking alcohol.
- You are in pain from an injury – always consult your practitioner first, as rest may be needed before you exercise.
- You have taken pain killers, as it will mask any warning pains.
- You are undergoing medical treatment, or are taking drugs – again, you will need to consult your medical practitioner first.

And remember, it is always wise to consult your doctor before you take up a new exercise regime. If you have a back problem you will need to consult your medical practitioner. Many of the exercises are wonderful for back-related problems, but you should always take expert guidance.

Please note that not all of the exercises are suitable for use during pregnancy, see page 235.

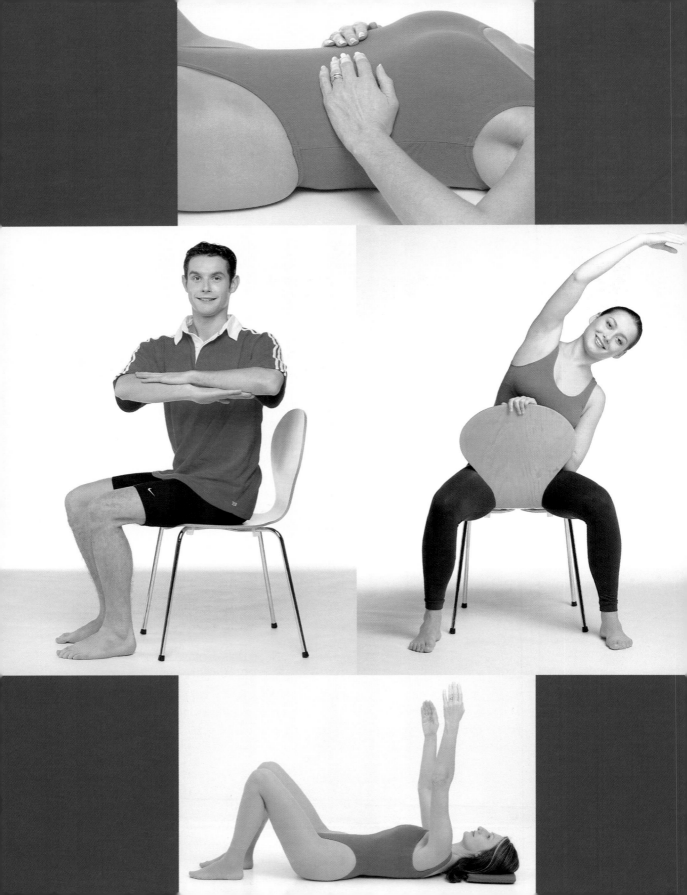

The
Beginner's
Programme

The exercises in this section will equip you with all the basic tools you need to learn how to move correctly. Once you have these skills, you may progress to the Intermediate Programme.

Relaxation Position

Equipment
A small flat firm pillow (optional).

Aim
To prepare the mind and the body for exercise. This position can also be used as a starting and finishing position for exercises and at the end of a session to unwind. It releases unwanted tension from the body, allowing the torso to widen and the spine to lengthen.

Starting Position
- Lie on a mat with a small firm flat pillow under your head. The idea is for the neck to be released and lengthened. You should feel very comfortable.
- Have your knees bent, place your feet in line with the hips. Some people are more comfortable with them placed a little wider, in line with the shoulders. This is fine. Keep your feet parallel. Your toes in the same line – initially you might need someone to check this for you.
- Place your hands on your abdomen.

Action
1 Allow your whole body to widen and lengthen.
2 Notice any areas of tension and allow them to melt gently into the floor.
3 Imagine that you have dry sand in your back pockets. Allow the sand to trickle slowly out of the pockets and onto the floor.
4 Release your thighs and soften the area round your hips.
5 Release your neck.

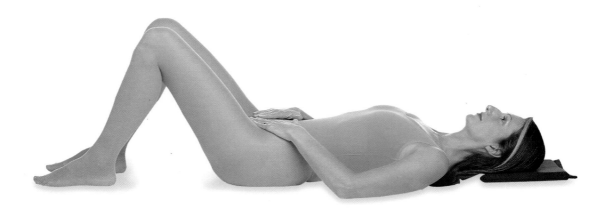

Lateral Breathing

With thoracic or lateral breathing, your lungs become like bellows, the lower ribcage expanding wide as you breathe in and closing down as you breathe out. This type of breathing encourages correct movement patterns by enabling you to stay centred while you move.

Equipment
A scarf or a towel.

Action
1 Sitting or standing tall wrap a scarf or towel round your ribs, crossing it over at the front.
2 Hold the ends of the scarf or towel. Keeping your shoulders relaxed, your elbows open. Pull it tight gently, breathe in wide and allow your ribs to expand the material.
3 As you breathe out allow the breastbone to soften. You may gently pull the scarf or towel in to help you empty your lungs fully and relax the ribcage. Repeat up to ten times. Watch that you keep your shoulders down and you do not lift the breastbone too high. Take natural easy breaths. Stop if you become dizzy.

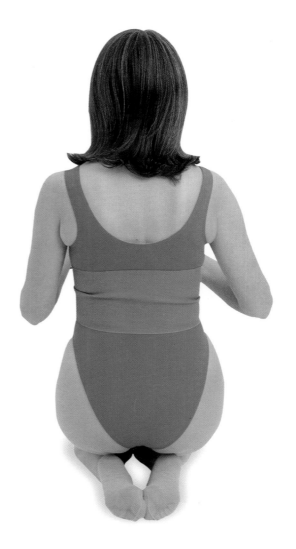

Breathing in the Relaxation Position

Aim

To combine lateral breathing with the Relaxation Position to encourage tension release and focus.

Starting Position

- Lie in the Relaxation Position – see page 28.

Action

1 Place your hands, on your lower ribcage.
2 Breathe in wide and full into your sides and into the floor, you should feel your fingers separate.
3 Breathe out and allow the ribs to close together gently.
4 Repeat eight gentle, but full, breaths.

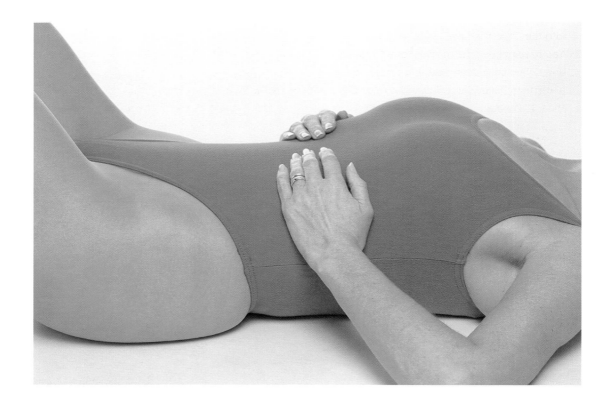

The Compass: Finding Neutral

Aim

To find the neutral position of the pelvis and spine.

Starting Position

- Lie in the Relaxation Position.
- Imagine that you have a compass on your lower abdomen, the navel is north, the pubic bone south, with west and east on either side.
- We are going to look at two incorrect positions in order to find the correct one.

Action

1 Tilt your pelvis up towards north – while doing so, the pelvis will 'tuck under'. Notice what has happened to your waist, your hips and your tailbone. The waist is flattened, you've pushed it into the floor, the curve of your low back is lost. You have gripped the muscles round your hips and tightened your six pack muscle (rectus abdominus), and your tailbone has lifted off the floor.

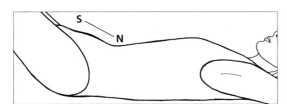

Tilted to north

2 Now, carefully (avoid this bit if you have a back injury), bring the pelvis so that it is tilting down towards south. Notice again what has happened. The low back is arched and feels vulnerable, your ribs have flared, you probably have two chins and your stomach is sticking out.

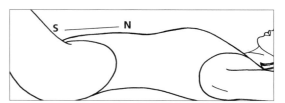

Tilted to south

3 Come back to the starting position.

We are aiming for a neutral position between the two extremes, neither to north nor to south, neither tucked nor arched. Back with the image of the compass, the pointer should be like a spirit level. The tailbone remains down on the floor and lengthens away. The pelvis keeps its length and is not 'scrunched up' at all. There remains a small natural arch in your back. This is neutral. All the exercises should be performed in this neutral position unless you are told otherwise. You should learn to recognize your natural neutral position when standing, lying, sitting or side-lying. You would not start your car if the gears were not in neutral, so please do not start an exercise! ▷

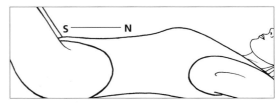

Neutral

Be particularly vigilant when you are engaging the lower abdominals (see page 32) as there is a temptation to tilt or tuck the pelvis. If you are lying down, you can always try placing your hand under your waist – you can feel if you are pushing the spine into the floor. You want to avoid this.

It is also worth pointing out that if you have a large bottom, you will have more of a hollow in the lumbar region – this does not necessarily mean that you have arched your back. Learn to recognize your natural curve.

Bear in mind, too, that the pelvis should also be level west to east. Many people suffer from a twisted pelvis. The pelvis can be rotated forward on one side as well as tilted. You need to be constantly aware that the pelvis stays neutral, level and stable while you exercise if the right muscles are to work. Of course, once we add movement into the programme the pelvis will sometimes move out of neutral, for example, in Roll Downs.

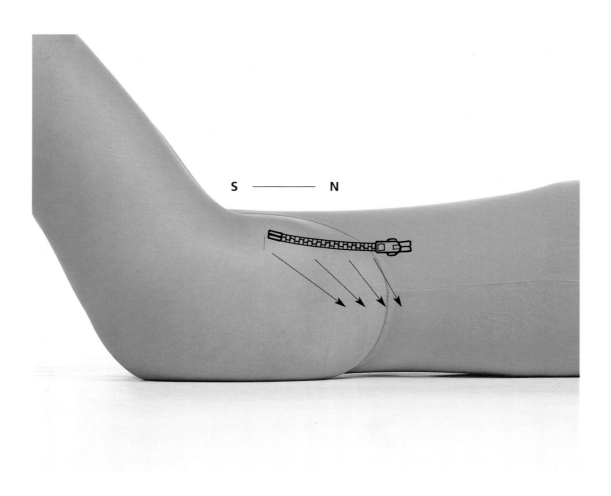

Lumbar Stabilization (Centring and Core Stability)

Aim

To isolate and engage the deep stabilizing muscles of the pelvis and spine – transversus abdominis, pelvic floor and multifidus muscles.

We have already discussed at length the importance of achieving core stability, of stabilizing the trunk, while we move. Clearly you also need to master engaging the deep stabilizing muscles before you begin the programme.

In order to achieve the best possible stability, you need to be able to contract the pelvic floor at the same time as hollowing the lower abdominals to engage transversus abdominis.

It is not easy to isolate and engage the pelvic floor muscles and it takes considerable concentration. We are talking about the urethra in men and women and the muscles of the vagina in women. At this stage we do not want you to engage the muscles round the anus, as it is too easy for the buttock muscles to kick in and substitute.

We know it sounds daft, but one way to help locate these muscles is to suck your thumb as you draw them up inside. Crazy, but effective! Otherwise, the following exercise should help you to find the right muscles and engage them at just the right percentage (30 per cent).

To engage these muscles correctly, think of:
- Hollowing
- Scooping
- Drawing the abdominals back towards the spine
- Sucking in ▷

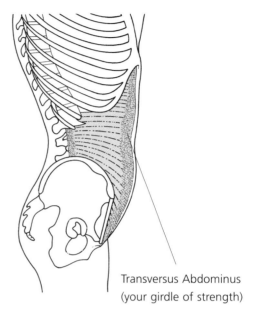

Transversus Abdominus
(your girdle of strength)

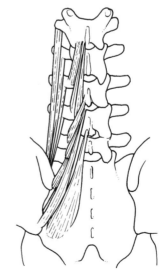

Multifidus

Sitting (The Pelvic Elevator)

Starting Position

- Sit on an upright chair.
- Make sure that you are sitting square with the weight evenly distributed on both buttocks.
- Imagine that your pelvic floor is like a lift in a building. This exercise requires you to take the lift up to different floors.

Action

1 Breathe in wide and full into your back and sides and lengthen up through the spine.
2 As you breathe out, draw up the muscles of your pelvic floor as if you were trying to prevent the flow of urine and take the pelvic lift up to the first floor of the building.
3 Breathe in and release the lift back to the ground floor.
4 Breathe out and now take the lift up to the second floor. Notice how when you do this the lower abdominals automatically engage.
5 Breathe in and release.
6 Breathe out and take the lift up to the third floor.
7 Breathe in and relax.

Watchpoints

- When you reached the second floor, you should have felt the deep lower abdominals engage. Although some people may feel this at the first floor. This is the transversus muscle coming into play. By starting the action from underneath, you encourage the 'six pack' muscle (rectus abdominis) to stay quiet. If you were to take the lift all the way to the top floor, you would probably be engaging the muscles at over 40 per cent and the rectus abdominis, which is a superficial abdominal muscle, would take over – so keep the action low and gentle

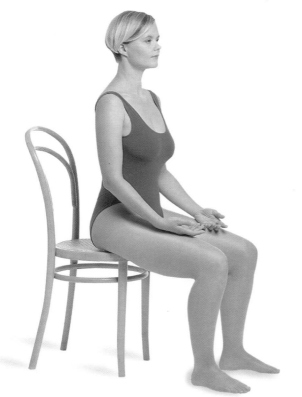

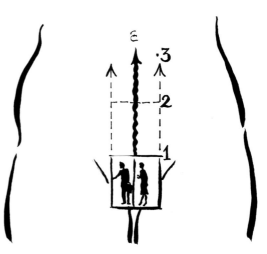

The pelvic elevator

- Do not allow the buttock muscles to join in.
- Keep your jaw relaxed.
- Don't take your shoulders up to the top floor too – keep them down and relaxed.
- Try not to grip round your hips.
- Keep the pelvis and spine quite still.

Once you have found your stabilizing muscles you need to learn how to engage them in lots of different positions. You should imagine your pelvic floor muscles as an internal zip which you zip up, hollowing the lower abdominals back to the spine. The instruction we will give you from now on will be 'zip up and hollow'.

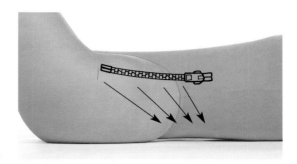

The following three positions will help to ensure that no cheating goes on.

Four Point Kneeling

Action

1 Kneel on all fours, your hands beneath your shoulders and shoulder-width apart.
2 Your knees are beneath your hips. Have the top of your head lengthening away from your tailbone. Your pelvis and spine are in neutral.

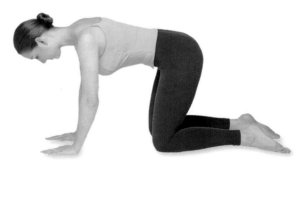

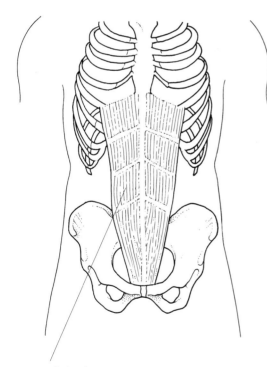

Rectus abdominus

The rectis abdminis (six-pack) muscle can become over-dominant

3 Breathe in to prepare.
4 Breathe out and zip up and hollow the lower abdominals up towards the spine. Your back should not move.
5 Breathe in and release. ▷

Prone lying

Action

1 Lie on your front. Rest your head on your folded hands, opening the shoulders out and relaxing the upper back – you may need a small, flat cushion under your abdomen if your low back is uncomfortable.
2 Your legs are shoulder-width apart and relaxed.
3 Breathe in to prepare, breathe out and zip up and hollow from the pelvic floor and lift the lower abdominals off the floor.
4 Imagine there is a precious egg under them that must not be crushed.
5 Do not tighten the buttocks.

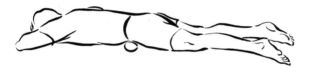

6 Breathe in and release.
7 Again there should be no movement in the pelvis or spine.

In the Relaxation Position (semi-supine)

Action

1 Lie on your back. Check that your pelvis is in neutral.
2 Breathe in to prepare and lengthen through the top of your head.

3 Breathe out and draw up the muscles of the pelvic floor and scoop the lower abdominals back towards the spine, hollowing out your lower stomach. Zip up and hollow.
4 Do not allow the pelvis to tuck under. Do not push into the spine. Keep your tailbone on the floor and lengthening away.
5 Breathe in and relax.

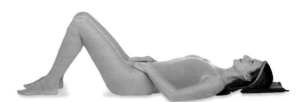

This, then, is your strong centre, and for most exercises, you will be asked to zip up and hollow, drawing the lower abdominals back to the spine, *before* and *while* you move, your movements lengthening away from this strong centre.

You must be careful not to tuck the pelvis under, that is tilting it to north. If you do, you will lose your neutral position and it means that other muscles – the rectus abdominis and the hip flexors – are cheating and doing the work instead of the transversus muscle. If you are comfortable with your hand under your waist you can check to see if you are pushing into the spine.

Note: Initially we teach zip and hollow on the out breath but once you have found the right muscles, you should keep them engaged for both the in and out breath.

Relaxation Position with Breathing and Stabilizing

Aim
To combine good alignment with lateral breathing and stabilizing.

Starting Position
- Lie in the Relaxation Position.

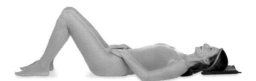

Action
1 Place your hands on your pelvis with the fingertips on the pubic bone and the heels of your hands resting on the pelvic bones. Check that your pubic bone and the pelvic bones are all level in your neutral pelvis position, neither tucked nor arched.

2 Move your hands to your lower ribcage and take a few deep breaths, breathing wide and full into your sides and into the floor. Think of breathing into the lower ribcage and the lungs expanding like bellows.

3 To find the deep postural muscles which stabilize your lumbar spine, breathe in and, as you breathe out, draw up the muscles of your pelvis and then zip up and hollow the lower abdominals back towards the spine. Do not tilt the pelvis at all, it remains completely still. Breathe in and release.

4 When you have mastered the lower ribcage breathing and you can zip up and hollow comfortably, try to maintain it while you *breathe in and out*. Make certain that your lower abdominals stay scooped and do not bulge at all.

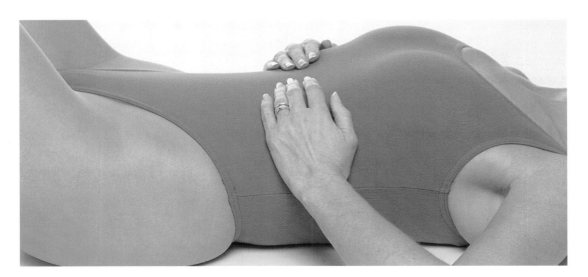

Pelvic Stability – Leg Slides, Drops, Folds and Turnout

Aim

To learn how to keep the pelvis in neutral and stable while the limbs are moved.

Now that you have mastered the breathing, the correct alignment of the pelvis and spine and the creation of a strong centre, isolating the stabilizing muscles, you need to learn how to add movement and how to co-ordinate all this. It isn't easy to begin with but, as with learning to ride a bicycle it soon becomes automatic. Meanwhile, the process of learning this co-ordination is fabulous mental and physical training as it stimulates that two-way communication between the brain and the muscles – real mind-body exercises.

We usually start with small, simple movements and then build up to more complicated combinations. Here we have given you four movements to practice, all of them requiring you to keep your pelvis completely still. A useful image is that a set of car headlamps is on your pelvis shining at the ceiling. The beam should be fixed and not mimicking searchlights! You can vary which exercises you practise at each session. The starting position is the same for all three.

Note: Notice that you are asked to zip and hollow before you move

Starting Position for Pelvic Stability exercises

- Adopt the Relaxation Position.
- Check that your pelvis is in neutral, tailbone down and lengthening away. Place your hands on your pelvic bones to check for unwanted movement and also check that the lower abdominals stay scooped and do not bulge.

Action for Leg Slides

1 Breathe in wide and full to prepare.
2 Breathe out, zip up and hollow and slide one leg away along the floor, keeping the lower abdominals engaged and the pelvis still, stable, and in neutral.
3 Breathe into your lower ribcage while you return the leg to the bent position, trying to keep the stomach hollow. If you cannot yet breathe in and maintain a strong centre, then take an extra breath and return the leg on the out breath.
4 Repeat five times with each leg.

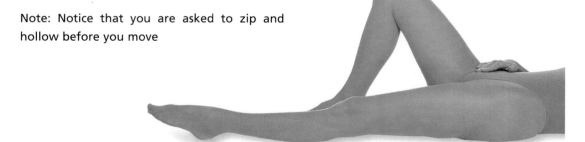

Leg slide: hands have been moved to show pelvic alignment

Action for Knee Drops

1 Breathe in wide and full to prepare.
2 Breathe out, zip up and hollow and allow one knee to open slowly to the side. Go only so far as the pelvis can remain still.
3 Breathe in, still zipped and hollowed, as the knee returns to centre.
4 Repeat five times with each leg, making sure that the pelvis does not roll to the side.

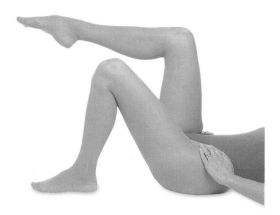

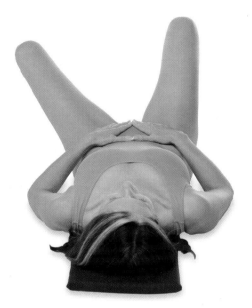

5 Repeat five times with each leg, making certain that your abdominals stay hollowed and scooped throughout. They must not bulge at all.

If you find that your abdominals bulge and/or your pelvis wobbles try imagining that you have bathroom scales under the foot you want to lift – as you try to lift the foot think about gradually taking your weight off the scales. You may not be able to lift the foot completely to start with but keep practising. Often one side is less stable than the other. ▷

Action for Knee Folds

1 Breathe in wide and full to prepare.
2 Breathe out, zip up and hollow and fold the right knee up. Think of the thigh bone dropping down into the hip and anchoring there. Do not lose your neutral pelvis, the tailbone stays down. Do not rely on the other leg to stabilize you. Imagine your foot is on a large chocolate cream eclair, you don't want to press down on it.
3 Breathe in and hold.
4 Breathe out, zipped and hollowed, as you return the foot slowly to the floor.

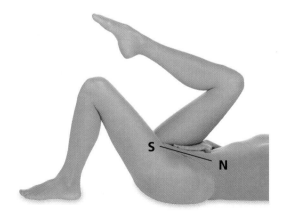

Incorrect Knee fold. The pelvis has tilted north

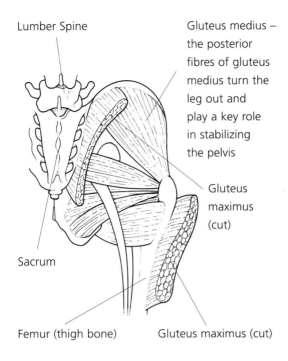

Lumber Spine

Gluteus medius –
the posterior
fibres of gluteus
medius turn the
leg out and
play a key role
in stabilizing
the pelvis

Gluteus
maximus
(cut)

Sacrum

Femur (thigh bone)   Gluteus maximus (cut)

The Pelvis (back view)

Action for Turning out the Leg

This next action involves turning the leg out from the hip. As you do so you are working your deep buttock muscles (gluteal muscles), especially gluteus medius which is one of the main stabilizing muscles of the pelvis.

Please take advice if you suffer from sciatica.

Follow steps 1 and 2 for Knee Folds page 39.

3 Breathe out, zip up and hollow and turn the right leg out from the hip bringing, if you can, the foot to touch the left knee. Do not allow the pelvis to tilt or twist or turn, keep it central and stable. Headlamps glued to the ceiling!

4 Breathe in and then out, zipped and hollowed, as you reverse the movement to return the foot to the floor.

5 Repeat five times to each side.

Watchpoints

* Remember that you are trying to avoid even the slightest movement of the pelvis. It helps to think of the waist being long and even on both sides as you make the movement.
* Try to keep your neck and jaw released throughout. If you feel tension creeping in, do a few Shoulder Drops (page 48) and Neck Rolls (page 50).
* Stay scooped.

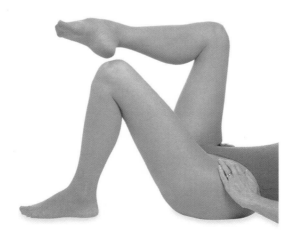

Turning out the leg

Good Upper Body Movement

Aim

We have been concentrating up until now on the lower half of the body. We also need to learn how to move the upper body correctly, with good technique. Remember that you need to maintain a strong centre while your arms move.

Look also at Floating Arms (page 58) and the Dart (page 70).

Starting Position

• Lie in the Relaxation Position, this time having your arms down by your sides.

Action

1 Breathe in wide into your lower ribcage to prepare.
2 Breathe out, zip up and hollow and start to take one arm back as if to touch the floor – you may not be able to touch the floor comfortably so only move the arm as far as you are happy to do so. Do not force the arm, keep it soft and open with the elbow bent. The shoulder blade stays down into your back. The ribs stay calm. Do not allow the back to arch at all.
3 Breathe in as you return the arms to your side.
4 Repeat five times with each arm.
5 Not everyone can touch the floor behind without arching the upper back. Do not strain. It is better to keep the back down than force the arm down.

Watchpoints

• Keep the arm quite wide it shouldn't end up close to your ear.
• Keep your elbow bent
• Keep the upper body open
• Keep the shoulder blade down into your back

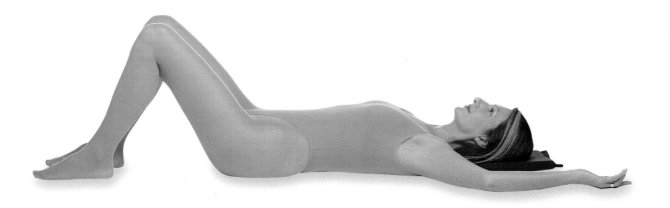

The Starfish

Aim

To establish good movement patterns throughout the body.

We are going to co-ordinate the opposite arm and leg. This is a sequence you first discovered when learning how to crawl as a child! Between the ages of four to seven months a child begins to learn to cross patterns, co-ordinating opposite arm and leg movement. This stage of development aids communication between the right and left hemi-spheres of the brain. Hopefully, everyone reading this will have mastered crawling, but as a neurolog-ical exercise it is helpful even for adults to practice and some of you may discover it isn't quite as easy as it sounds!

Starting Position

• As for Good Body Movement.

Action

1 Breathe in wide and full to prepare.
2 Breathe out, zip up and hollow and slide the left leg away along the floor and take the right arm above you in a backstroke movement. Keep the pelvis completely neutral, stable and still, and the stomach muscles engaged. Keep a sense of width and openness in the upper body and shoulders, and try to keep the shoulder blades down into your back.
3 Breathe in, still zipped and hollowed, and return the limbs to the starting position.
4 Repeat five times, alternating arms and legs.

These may not seem like difficult movements but to do them properly takes great concentration and skill. You are basically trying to re-train your muscle recruitment, so please do not be tempted to skip learning these basic skills as they are invaluable in mastering the more difficult exercises.

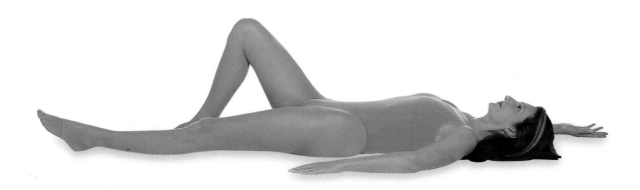

Knee Stirs

Aim

To release the muscles round the hip, promote hip mobility and pelvic stability.

If you sit all day at a desk, there is a possibility that the muscles round the hips become very tight. Strangely enough the other group of people who tend to have dominant hip flexors are fitness enthusiasts – frequently the hip flexors become overly strong as they substitute for the transversus muscle in abdominal exercises.

This is a lovely exercise for helping those muscles to release. It also takes the hip joint through a range of movement that is not usual in everyday life – thus helping to ensure that the ability to make the movement is kept. At the same time, the exercise will help promote lubrication of the joint. If all this hasn't convinced you yet, try it and enjoy the sense of release it gives.

Starting Position

- Lie in the Relaxation Position.
- Wrap a scarf round one thigh, holding it from underneath so that the shoulders stay down and relaxed.
- Fold the knee up, so that it is directly above the hip.

Action

1 Keeping the pelvis neutral and stable – that is, not allowing it to rock from side to side – gently and slowly circle the bent leg.
2 Breathe normally as you do so, zipping and hollowing throughout. Think of releasing the thigh bone from the hip socket. Allow the scarf (and your hands) to help move the leg.
3 Circle five times clockwise and five times anti-clockwise with each leg.

Moving on . . .

Once you can recognize that feeling of release round the joint, combined with a strong centre and a stable pelvis, you may try the exercise without the scarf.

Watchpoints

- Check that holding the scarf hasn't created tension in the upper body. If it has, try the exercise without the scarf while maintaining the sense of openness.
- Keep checking that your pelvis is in neutral, tailbone down and lengthening away.
- Don't take the leg too wide to begin with – initially the circle should be the size of a grapefruit. You may take it wider as you become more confident.

Ankle Circles

Aim

To free the ankle joint, increasing its mobility. To work the muscles, ligaments and tendons surrounding the ankle joint. To work the calf muscles.

For many of us, the muscles on the outer side of the ankle tend to be weak, which is why we are prone to sprained ankles as you 'roll over' on the outside of the foot. This exercise is great for strengthening them.

Starting Position

- Lie on your back in the Relaxation Position.
- Bend one knee up and take hold of it just behind the knee, with your thumbs coming round in front of it – this is so that you can feel if your leg is moving.

Action

1 Start to circle the foot very, very slowly and, taking it as far as you can, go to the maximum. The leg should stay completely still, the movement coming totally from the ankle joint. Do not just wiggle your toes round.

2 Do five circles each way.

Watchpoints

- What was happening to the rest of your body? Remember, shoulder blades down, breastbone soft, elbows open, lateral breathing, neutral pelvis.
- You do not need to zip up and hollow throughout this exercise, so use this as a break from stabilizing.

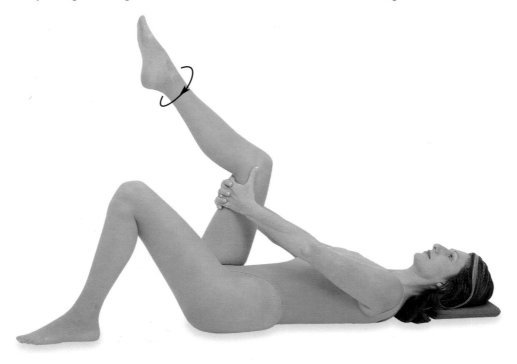

Spine Curls

Aim

To learn segmental control of the spine at an inter-vertebral level and to gain the ability to 'wheel' the spine, vertebra by vertebra promoting flexibility and stability throughout its length.

In a healthy back all the different segments of the spine work together to create the desired movement, each vertebra contributing to that movement – a bit like a bicycle chain. When one level is locked, the movement of the chain is upset. What often happens is that the levels above and below the locked area become over-flexible to compensate for the area that will not move – you can be hypo-mobile (not enough movement) in one area and hyper-mobile (too much movement) above and/or below. This puts enormous strain on the back.

Many Pilates exercises work towards this goal of promoting flexibility and stability, exercises such as this and Roll Downs on page 92 encourage this segmental control.

Joseph Pilates referred to this way of moving as 'using the spine like a wheel' ▷

The Cervical Spine: the most mobile of all the spinal areas permitting all movements.

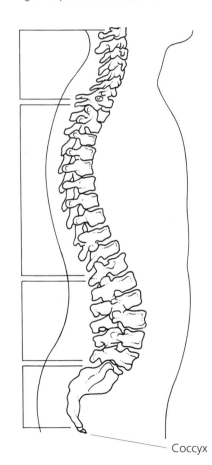

The Thoracic Spine: this is the least mobile of all the spinal areas due to the attachment of the ribs. There is little ability to bend forward or backward, but if you wish to twist or rotate, most of the action will take place here, especially in the section just above the hollow of your back.

The Lumbar Spine: here, rotation is very limited, but forward and backward bending (flexion and extension) occur mainly from this area.

Sacrum

The movement potential of your spine may depend on your posture

Coccyx

Starting Position

- Lie in the Relaxation Position, your feet about 20 centimetres from your buttocks, hip-width apart and parallel.
- Plant the feet firmly on the floor.
- *If it is comfortable*, take your arms above your head and rest them on the floor, keeping them wider than shoulder-width, relaxed and open – your upper back must not be arched.
- Otherwise, leave your arms down by your sides, palms down.

Action

1 Breathe in wide and full to prepare.
2 Breathe out, zip up and hollow and slowly and carefully curl just the base of your spine (tailbone) off the floor – you will lose the neutral pelvis position.
3 Breathe in and breathe out, still zipping up and hollowing, as you lower and lengthen the spine back onto the floor.
4 Repeat, lifting a little more of the spine off the floor each time. As you lower, put down each part of the spine in sequence, bone by bone. Aim to put 'three inches' between each vertebra, the back of the ribs, the waist, the small of the back, the tailbone.
5 You should complete five full curls, wheeling and lengthening the spine.

Watchpoints

- Take care that your back does not arch and that your tailbone stays tucked under like a whippet who has just been told off!
- Do not curl up too high – just to the level of your shoulder blades.
- Do not rush the first few curls. Really make the base of the spine move.
- There is a tendency sometimes, when there is a muscle imbalance in the torso, for one side to dominate. If you think of the spine landing like a jet on a runway, it would look as though you were landing in a high cross wind! Try to land down the central strip of the runway – no cross winds!!!
- Keep the pressure through your feet equal.

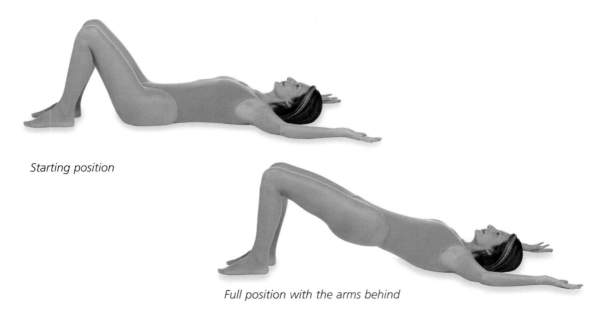

Starting position

Full position with the arms behind

Hip Flexor Stretch

Aim

To lengthen the hip flexors gently.

If you sit all day, it is likely that your hip flexor muscles will shorten. If they do, this will affect the angle of your pelvis pulling it forward anteriorly.

Starting Position

- Lie in the Relaxation Position page 28.

Action

1 Breathe in wide and full to prepare.
2 Breathe out, zip up and hollow, bend the right knee up to your chest, dropping the thigh bone down into the hip joint.
3 Breathe in, as you clasp the right leg below the knee or round the lower part of the thigh. If you have any knee problems clasp the leg under the thigh rather than below the knee so that the joint is not compressed.

4 Breathe out, still zipping and hollowing and stretch the left leg along the floor. Your lower back should remain in neutral. If it arches, bend the left knee back up again a little. Hold this stretch for five breaths.
5 On your next breath, still zipped, slide the leg back.
6 Breathe in and then out out as you lower the right leg back to the floor, keeping the abdominals engaged.
7 Repeat twice on each side, keeping your shoulders relaxed and down.

Watchpoints

- Check the position of the upper body, elbows open, breastbone soft, shoulder blades down into the back, neck released.
- Are you in neutral?

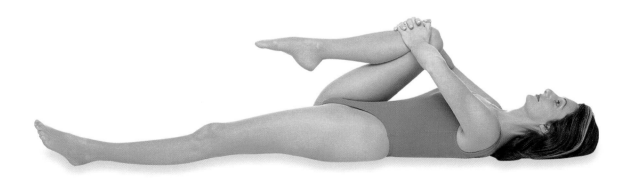

Shoulder Drops and Cross Over Shoulder Drops

Aim

To release tension in the upper body.

A wonderful exercise that allows you to let go of any tension round the shoulders and neck. Great to do at the end of a stress-filled day.

Starting Position

- Lie in the Relaxation Position page 28.

Action

1 Raise both arms towards the ceiling directly above your shoulders, palms facing each other.

2 Breathe in wide and full and reach up to the ceiling with one arm and stretch up through the fingertips. The shoulder blade comes off the floor. As you breathe out drop the shoulder back down onto the floor.

3 Repeat ten times with each arm. Feel your upper back widening and the tension in your shoulders releasing down into the floor.

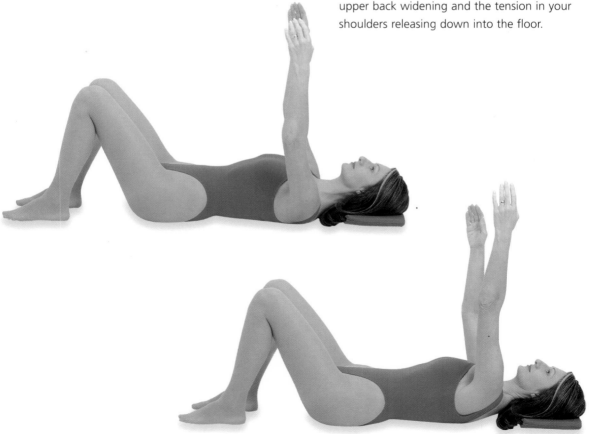

Cross Over Shoulder Drops

When you are comfortable with the above, try this variation. You will need to keep the pelvis stable for this version, which means adding the zip up and hollow.

Starting Position

• As above.

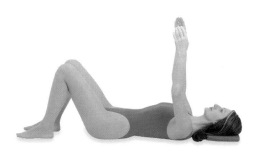

Action

1 Breathe in wide and full to prepare.
2 Breathe out, zip up and hollow, keeping the pelvis still and square. Reach one hand up across the other to where the ceiling meets the wall. Your shoulder blade will leave the floor, your head should move gently with you. Enjoy the stretch between the shoulder blades.
3 Breath in and hold the stretch.
4 Breathe out and relax the shoulder back down to the floor.
5 Repeat ten times to each side, making sure that the pelvis stays quite still.

Watchpoints

• Whichever version you are doing, keep the distance between the ears and the shoulders.
• The shoulder blade leaves the floor, but should stay down toward toward your waist.

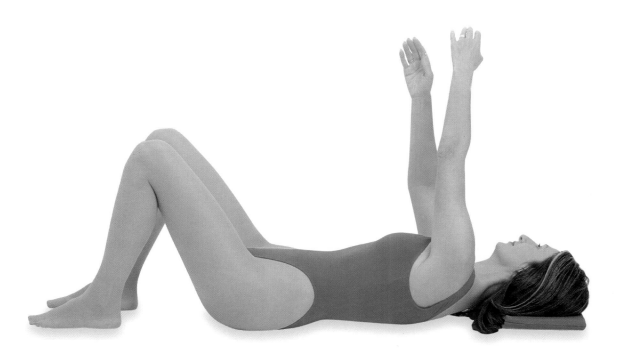

Neck Rolls and Chin Tucks

Aim

To release tension from the neck, freeing the cervical spine. To use the deep stabilizers of the neck, deep neck flexors. To lengthen the neck extensors.

Another important aspect in re-educating the head-neck relationship lies in the relative strength of the neck extensors (those which tilt the head back) and flexors (those which tilt the head forward). If you think about how we sit at a desk or the steering wheel, we usually have our head thrust forward and tipped back so there is a muscle imbalance. We need to release the superficial neck flexors and engage the deep neck flexors. By relaxing the jaw,

lengthening the back of the neck and tucking the chin in gently, we can redress the balance.

Please take note that we want you to tuck the chin in gently, nothing too vicious, it is a subtle movement.

Starting Position

- Lie in the Relaxation Position, with your knees bent and your arms resting on your lower abdomen.
- Only use a flat pillow for this if you are uncomfortable without, your head will roll better if you do not use one.

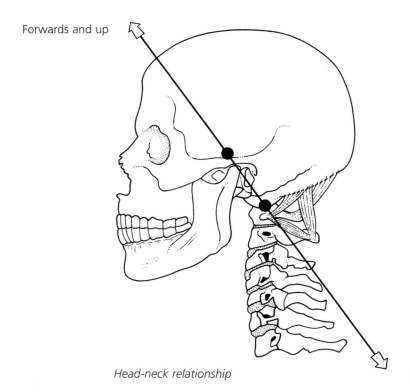

Forwards and up

Head-neck relationship

Back and down

Action

1 Release your neck, release your jaw, allow your tongue to widen at its base. Keep the neck nicely lengthened. Soften your breastbone and allow the shoulder blades to widen and melt into the floor.

2 Now, allow your head to roll slowly to one side.

3 Bring it back to the centre and over to the other side. Just let the head roll slowly from side to side, do not rush, take your time.

4 When the neck feels free bring the head to the centre and gently tuck your chin in, keeping the head on the floor and lengthening out of the back of the neck. It is subtle movement – imagine you need to hold a ripe peach under the chin – you do not wish to crush its fragile skin.

5 Return the head to the centre.

6 Repeat the rolling to the side and chin tuck eight times.

Watchpoints

• Do not force the head or neck, just let it roll naturally.

• Do not lift the head off the floor when you tuck the chin in.

• If you find your jaw becomes tense as you tuck your chin in, gently place the tip of your tongue on the roof of your mouth behind your front teeth as you lengthen through the back of the neck.

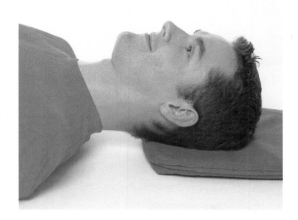

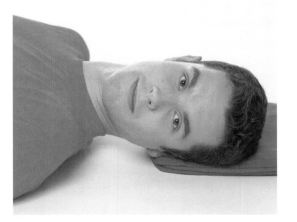

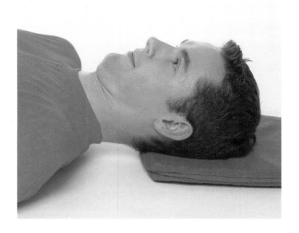

Arm Openings

Equipment
A bedroom pillow, and a tennis ball (optional).

Aim
To open the upper body and stretch the pectoral muscles, while stabilizing the shoulder blades. To achieve a sense of openness while stabilizing and centring. To rotate the spine gently and safely.

This has to be the most relaxing, feel good exercise in the Pilates programme. Stay completely aware of your arm and hand as it displaces the air while moving through space.

Please note that as this exercise involves rotation of the spine, you should take advice if you have a disc-related injury.

Starting Position
- Lie on your side, your head on a pillow, knees curled up at a right angle to your body. Your back should be in a straight line, but keeping its natural curve.
- Place a tennis ball between the knees (the idea is for the tennis ball to keep your knees and pelvis in good alignment). Line all your bones up on top of each other: feet, ankles, knees, hips and shoulders.
- Your arms are extended in front of you, your palms together at shoulder height.

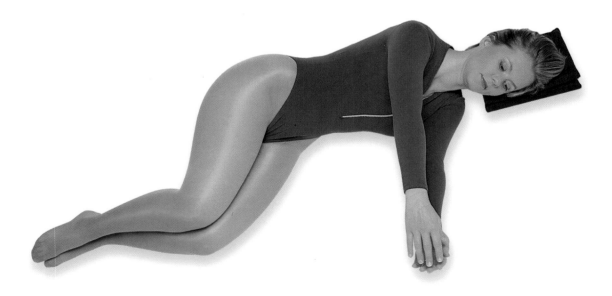

Action

1 Breathe in to prepare and lengthen through the spine.

1 Breathe out and zip up and hollow.

2 Breathe in as you slowly extend and lift the upper arm, keeping the elbow soft and the shoulder blade down into the back. Keep your eyes on your hand so that the head follows the arm movement. You are aiming to touch the floor behind your back, but do not force it. Try to keep your knees together, your pelvis still. Stay zipped and hollowed.

4 Breathe out as you bring the arm back in an arc to rest on the other hand again.

5 Repeat five times, then curl up on the other side and start again.

Watchpoints

• Keep hollowing throughout.

• Keep your waist long, don't allow it to sink into the floor.

• Don't forget to allow your head to roll naturally with the movement, make sure that it is supported by the pillow.

• Keep the gap between your ears and your shoulders by engaging the muscles below the shoulder blades.

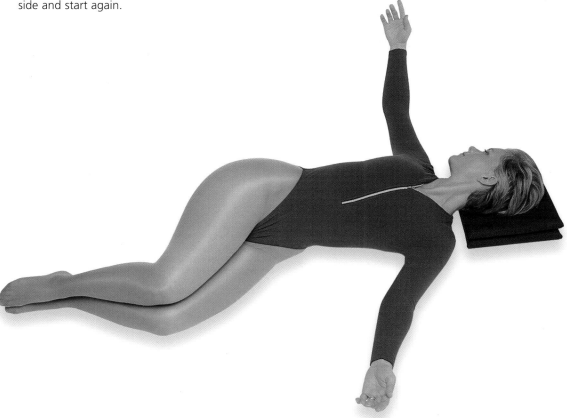

Side Rolls

Aim

To achieve rotation of the spine with stability. To work the waist muscles (obliques).

Starting Position

- Lie in the Relaxation Position, feet hip-width apart and in parallel.
- Place your arms palms up out to the sides at shoulder height alongside your body. Allow the floor to support you.
- Allow your body to widen and lengthen.

Action

1 Breathe in wide and full to prepare.
2 Breathe out, zip up and hollow, roll your head in one direction, your knees in the other. Only roll a little way to start with – you can go further each time if it is comfortable. Keep your opposite shoulder down on the floor.
3 Breathe in, still zipping and hollowing.
4 Breathe out, use your strong centre to bring the knees back to the starting position. Bring the head back to the starting position as well.
5 Repeat eight times in each direction. Think of rolling each part of your back off the floor in sequence and then returning the back of the ribcage, the waist, the small of your back, the buttock to the floor.

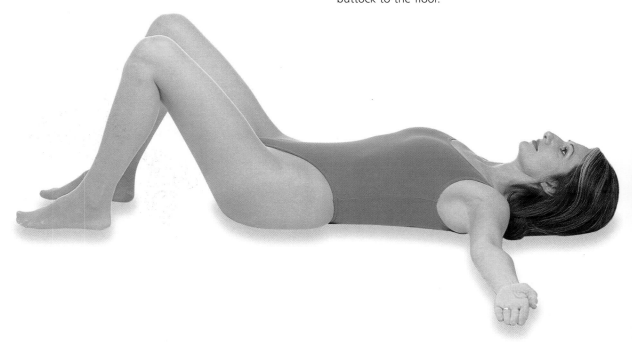

Starting position

Moving on . . . .

Try the same exercise, but this time bring the feet together and place a tennis ball between the knees. It is performed in exactly the same way as before, but keeping the tennis ball between the knees means that the pelvis stays in good alignment. It also means that you have to work the waist that bit harder to stay in line.

Watchpoints

- Keep the pelvis in neutral, taking care that you do not allow it to arch.
- Keep working those abdominals. Do not simply allow the weight of the legs to pull you.

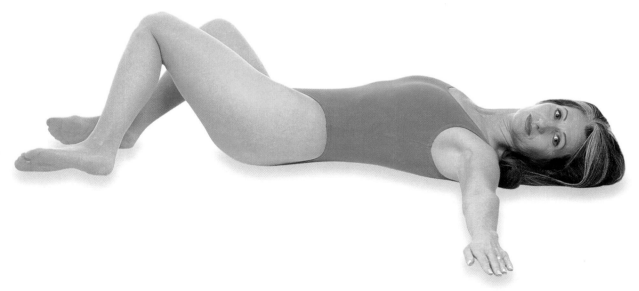

Full position

Standing Correctly and The Dumb Waiter

Aim

To become aware of the shoulder blades and of their relationship with the ribcage. To open the chest, especially the front of the upper arms/shoulders. To strengthen the weak external rotator muscles of the shoulder joint (those that turn the shoulder joint outwards). All this to be done with the shoulder blades set down into the back, stabilized.

Starting Position

- This exercise can be done anywhere, standing or sitting on a chair.

Standing Well

Imagine your head as effortlessly balancing on top of your spine.

Allow your shoulder blades to rest down into your back

Let your tailbone gently drop towards the floor as if you had a weight attached to it, but still maintaining the natural neutral spine/pelvis position (see page 31)

Relax your weight through the bones of the skeleton, working with gravity

Stand comfortably with your feet hip-width apart, your feet parallel

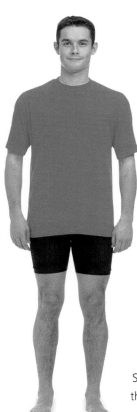

Release your head upwards, towards the ceiling, and lengthen the spine. Imagine balloons on a string attached to the top of your head lifting you up

Let your arms hang comfortably by your side

Gently zip up and hollow, engaging the pelvic floor and hollowing out the lower abdominals

Gently release your knees, unlocking them

Spread your feet on the floor, distributing the weight evenly. Imagine a triangle from the base of the big toe, the base of the little toe and the centre of the heel

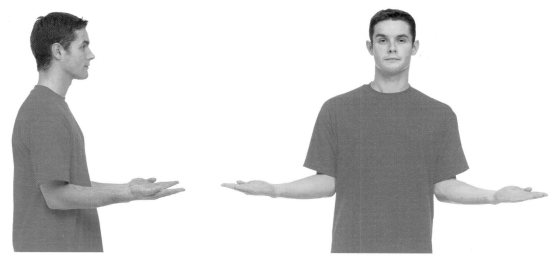

Starting position

Full position

- If you choose to sit, sit well forward on the chair with your pelvis in neutral and, your feet planted on the floor hip-width apart, your weight even on both buttocks! Hold your arms, palms facing upwards, your elbows tucked into your waist.
- If you wish to stand, follow the directions given.

Action

1 Breathe in to prepare and lengthen up through the spine.
2 Breathe out, zip up and hollow.
3 Breathe in, still zipping and hollowing and keeping your elbows into your sides, take your hands backwards, opening them, and working the muscles between the shoulder blades. Keep the shoulder blades down.
4 Breathe out and return the hands to the starting position.
5 Repeat five times.

Watchpoints

- Do not allow the upper back to arch as you take the arms back.
- If you find this very easy, check that your elbows are staying in and your shoulder blades staying down.
- Keep your neck released.

Floating Arms (Standing)

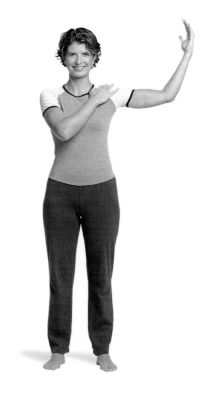

Aim
To practice correct shoulder movement, stabilizing the shoulder blades by using the lower trapezius and serratus anterior. We are aiming to minimize the workload of the upper trapezius which tends to be overworked which can cause great tension in the neck and shoulders – see page 259 on Shoulder Problems.

Starting Position
Standing comfortably, follow directions on page 56.

Action
1 Now place your right hand on your left shoulder, your left arm is hanging by your side, the palm angled, facing forward.
2 Breathe in to prepare and lengthen up through the spine, letting the neck be free.

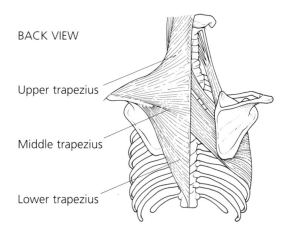

BACK VIEW

Upper trapezius

Middle trapezius

Lower trapezius

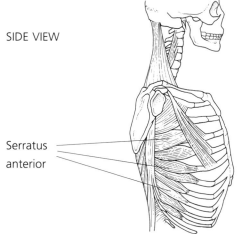

SIDE VIEW

Serratus anterior

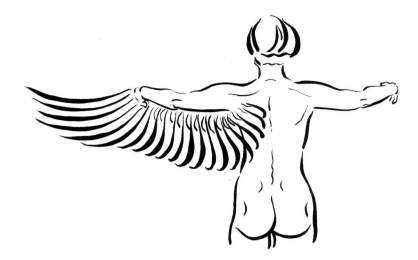

3 Breathe out, zip up and hollow and slowly begin to raise the arm reaching wide out of the shoulder blades like a bird's wing. Think of the hand as leading the arm, the arm following the hand as it floats upwards. You will need to rotate the arm so that the palm opens to the ceiling as the arm reaches shoulder level. Try to keep the shoulder under your hand as still as possible with the shoulder blades dropping down into your back as long as possible.

4 Breathe in as you lower the arms to your side.

5 Repeat three times with each arm.

Watchpoints

• Keep a sense of openness in the upper body.
• Do not allow your upper body to shift to the side, keep central.

Moving on . . .

As soon as you feel that you have mastered keeping the shoulders down while raising the arm and using the shoulder blades correctly, you can try raising both arms together. You may need the help of a mirror to check that you are doing it correctly.

Take care when raising both arms that you do not allow the upper body to sway backwards. If you find that you are swaying, do not raise the arms so high.

Pole Raises

Aim

To learn correct upper-body use. To open the upper body, gently stretching the pectorals and upper arms/shoulders (anterior deltoids).

Practise Floating Shoulders before attempting this exercise.

Equipment

A light, strong but flexible, pole or a scarf or thera-band (a stretch band) approximately 1.5 to 1.8 metres long.

Starting Position

- Stand correctly. Lengthening through the spine.
- Hold the pole lightly with both hands, about one metre apart.

Action

1 Breathe in wide and full to prepare.
2 Breathe out and zip up and hollow as you raise the pole, allowing the movement of the hands and the pole to lead the arms and shoulders. Try to keep the upper shoulders relaxed – don't let them hike up round your ears. Think of the shoulder blades dropping down as the arms rise. Make the movement initiate from your shoulder blades.
3 Breathe in.
4 Breathe out as you bring the pole onto your forehead, bringing the shoulder blades down into your back as you do so.
5 Breathe in and raise the pole.
6 Breathe out and slowly lower the pole, again using those muscles below the shoulder blades.
7 Repeat five times.

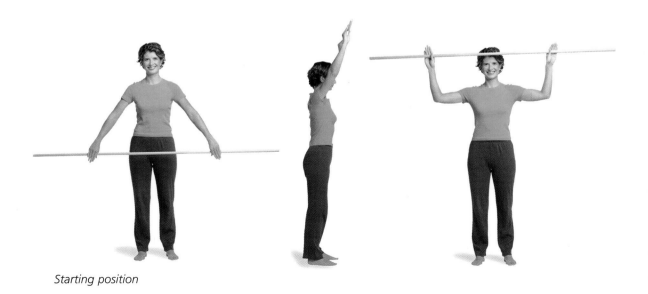

Starting position

Moving on . . .

When you are comfortable with this movement, follow directions 1–3 then:

4 Breathe out and bring the pole directly down behind you, keeping it close to your body and bending the elbows, so that you have a chicken-wing shape. Think of the shoulder blades drawing down and together.

5 Breathe in as you raise the pole slowly from behind and breathe out as you bring it slowly back down in front.

6 Repeat up to five times.

Watchpoints

- Do not allow the back to arch – keep the neutral spine alignment.
- Try not to duck your head as the pole comes over.
- Try to keep both shoulders and arms moving together, don't allow one shoulder to dominate.
- Keep reminding yourself of the standing instructions (page 56), lengthening the spine upwards.

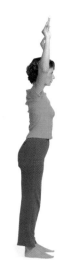

Incorrect

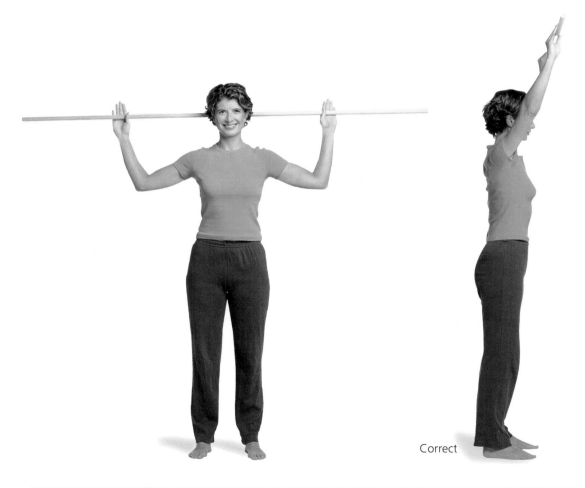

Correct

The Cossack and Waist Twist

Aim

To learn rotation of the spine with stability and length.

Please consult your practitioner before doing this exercise if you have a disc-related injury.

Starting Position

- Sit on a chair, your feet firmly planted hip-width apart on the floor.
- Fold your arms in front of you, in line with your chest or just below if this is more comfortable.
- Keep the shoulders down and your neck soft.

Action

1 Breathe in and lengthen up through your spine.
2 Breathe out, zip up and hollow and turn to the right as far as you can while keeping your pelvis square and forward facing.
3 Breathe in to lengthen up, still zipping and hollowing and return to the front.
4 Repeat five times to each side. Remember to keep lengthening up.

Watchpoints

- Do not allow the shoulders to creep up round the ears. Keep the shoulder blades down into the back.
- Try to keep the weight evenly balanced on both buttocks and also on both feet.
- Do not turn the head too far. It should move naturally, balanced on top of the spine.
- Try not to tilt forward with one shoulder, stay central.

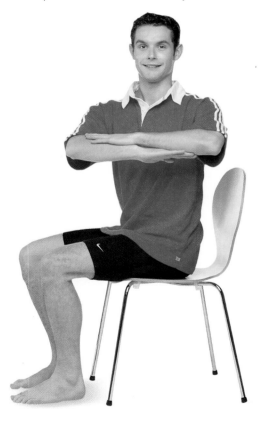

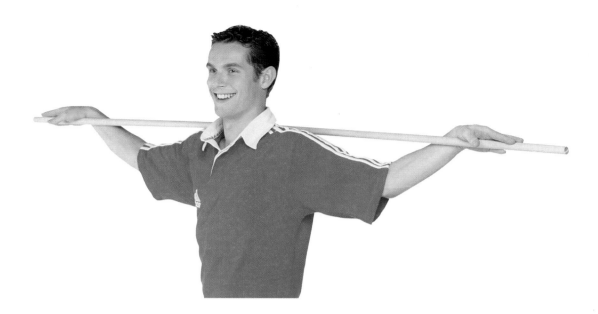

Moving On . . .

Standing Waist Twists

Equipment

A strong pole about 1.5 to 1.8 metres in length. A thick bamboo pole is ideal as it retains some flexibility.

Starting Position

Place the pole across your shoulders, taking your arms round and under with your hands resting on the pole. If this is too uncomfortable, hold your arms out to the side. If they tire, lower them as necessary.

Action

1 Breathe in as you lengthen up through the spine.
2 Breathe out, zip up and hollow and, keeping your pelvis square and facing forward, gently turn your upper body round as far as is comfortable. Your head will turn also. Only turn as far as you can keep your pelvis square and still.
3 Breathe in as you return to centre.
4 Repeat up to ten times to each side.

Watchpoints

- As for the previous exercise, but you will have to work harder and pay close attention to keeping the correct pelvic alignment.
- If you find your pelvis moving, stand in front of a table or the back of a chair with your thighs just touching it – this gives you an idea of when you twist the pelvis.

Side Reaches (Sitting and Standing)

Sitting

Aim

To stretch the sides, especially the waist (quadratus lumborum) muscles, while achieving a sense of lengthening and stability. To learn shoulder blade stabilization.

Equipment

A sturdy chair.

Starting Position

• You'll need to turn your chair round for this one. If you can, sit astride the chair, holding on to the backrest, both sitting bones (ischia) firmly planted on the chair, your feet flat on the ground.

Action

1 Breathe in wide and full to prepare, breathe out and raise one hand over your head, the palm facing downward, the shoulder staying down into the back.
2 Breathe in and lengthen up through the spine.
3 Breathe out, zip up and hollow, as you slowly reach across to the top corner of the room. Keep your bottom firmly planted while you lift out of the hips. Do not arch your lower back, keep your head and neck in line with the spine.
4 Breathe in and return to centre, lower the arm.
5 Change hands and repeat on the other side.
6 Repeat five times to each side, making sure that you go directly to the side as if moving between two sliding doors.

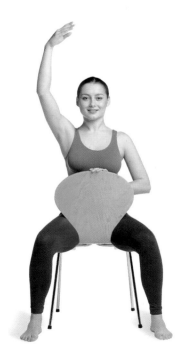
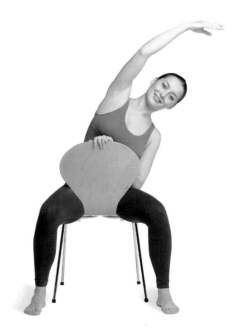

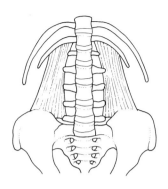

Quadratus Lumborum

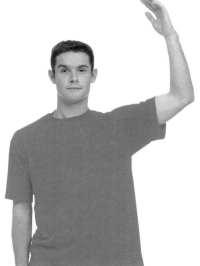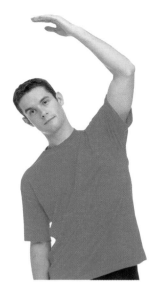

Standing

Try the same exercise now in a standing position.

Starting Position
- Stand with your feet wider than your hips. Have your knees slightly bent and remember all the standing directions (page 56).
- Your arms are down by your side resting on your thighs.

Action
1 Breathe in and lengthen up through the spine as you raise one arm up, keep your shoulder blade down into your back for as long as possible and keep your neck and upper shoulders soft.
2 Breathe out, zip up and hollow. Lengthening upwards you are going to reach towards the opposite top corner of the room. Your other arm slides down the outside of the thigh. Feel the distance increase between your ribcage and your pelvis. Make sure that you go directly to the side and not forward or backward. Keep your focus ahead and do not look down or up.
3 Breathe in and keep lengthening upwards.
4 Breathe out, still zipped and hollowed, and slowly return to upright and then lower the arm.
5 Repeat five times to each side.

Watchpoints
- Be careful not just to bend sideways collapsing the waist, you must keep lengthening upwards.
- You must stay in line. Imagine that you are sliding between two walls.
- Keep the other arm on your leg, it will slide downwards as you bend.
- Watch the angle of your head – you want to keep the head on top of the spine, looking forwards. If you look down, you have lost that head-neck relationship.
- Keep your pelvis central.

Sliding down the Wall

Aim

To learn how to lengthen the base of the spine, achieving the correct angle of the pelvis to the spine. Works the thigh muscles and stretches the Achilles tendon.

This exercise has the advantage that it can be practised anywhere, even where space is limited – during an aeroplane flight, for example.

To achieve good posture it is essential that the pelvis is at the correct angle to the spine. This is a wonderful way to learn to lengthen the base of the spine but without over-tilting the pelvis, or tucking under too far. Always remember 'north to south'.

If you have back problems it is vital that the thigh muscles stay strong so that you may bend your knees and squat while you lift heavy objects!

Starting Position

- Stand with your back to the wall and your feet about 15 centimetres away from the wall.
- Your feet are hip-width apart and parallel.
- Lean back into the wall. Don't try to force your head back onto the wall, just stand comfortably.
- Before you begin, take note which parts of your back are touching the wall.

Action

1 Breathe in wide and full to prepare, lengthening through the spine.
2 Breathe out, zip up and hollow, bend your knees and slide about 30 centimetres down the wall until your thighs are almost parallel with the floor – don't go any lower than this! Keep

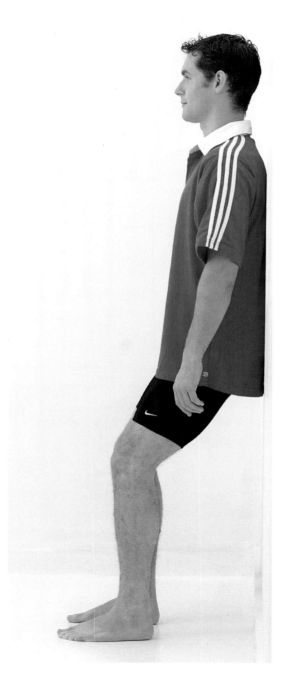

your feet flat on the floor (your heels will want to come up – don't let them). Don't allow your tailbone to lift off the wall, rather keep it lengthening away from you.

3 Breathe in as you slide back up, still zipping and hollowing and trying to keep the base of the spine lengthened.

4 Repeat eight times.

5 As you leave the wall, stand upright for a moment imagining that the wall is still there.

Watchpoints

- Watch that you don't slide down too far – never take your bottom below knee level.
- Check that your knees are passing directly over your feet and not inside them. Your feet must stay parallel, don't let them roll inwards.
- Keep your heels on the floor.
- Remember, do not let your tailbone lift off the wall!

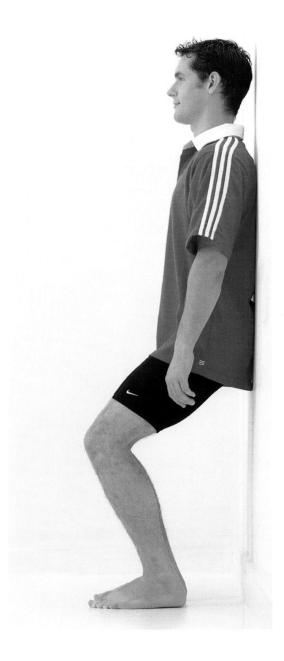

Roll Downs

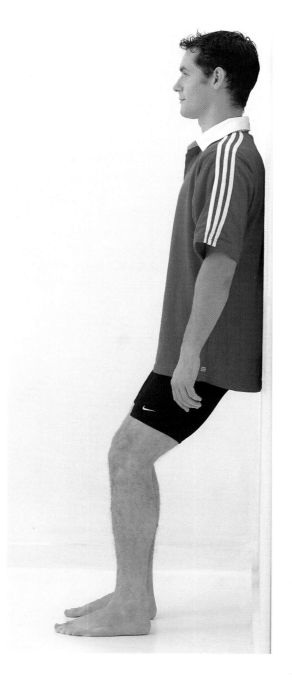

Aim

To release tension in the spine, the shoulders and the upper body. To mobilize the spine, creating flexibility and strength and achieving segmental control. To teach correct use of stabilizing abdominals when bending.

This is a core exercise in any Pilates programme, it can be used as a warm up or a wind down. It combines stabilizing work with the wonderful wheeling motion of the spine. As you roll back up, think of rebuilding the spinal column, stacking each vertebra one on top of the other to lengthen out the spine.

Please take advice if you have a back problem (see below), especially disc-related.

Starting Position

- Stand about 45 centimetres from a wall (the distance really depends on your height, but you should feel comfortable).
- Your knees are bent so that from the side you look as if you are sitting on a bar stool! Have your feet hip-width apart and in parallel with your weight evenly balanced on both feet. Check that you are not rolling your feet in or out.
- Find your neutral pelvis position but keep the tailbone lengthening down.

Action

1 Breathe in to prepare and lengthen up through the spine, release the head and neck.
2 Breathe out, zip up and hollow, drop your chin onto your chest and allow the weight of your head to make you roll slowly forward, head released, arms hanging, centre strong, knees

soft. If you have a back problem, you may like to begin by sliding your hands down your thighs.

3 Breathe in as you hang, really letting your head and arms hang.

4 Breathe out, firmly zipped up and hollowed, as you drop your tailbone down, directing your pubic bone forward, rotating your pelvis backwards as you slowly come up the wall, rolling through the spine bone by bone.

5 Repeat six times.

Watchpoints

- You may like to take an extra breath during the exercise. This is fine, but please try to breathe out as you move the spine.
- Make sure that you go down centrally and do not sway over to one side. When you are down, check where your hands are in relation to your feet.
- Do not roll the feet in or out. Keep the weight evenly balanced and try not to lean forward onto the front of your feet or back onto the heels.

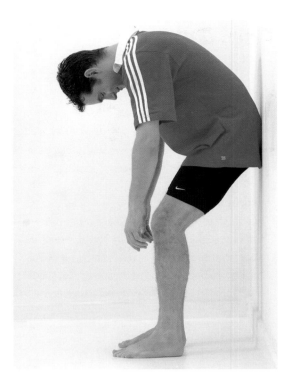

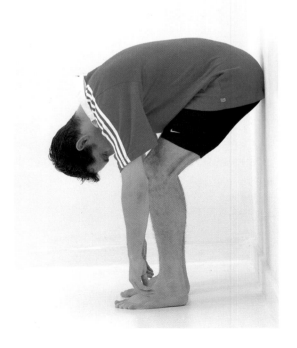

The Dart

Aim

To strengthen the back extensor muscles with trunk stability. To create awareness of the shoulder blades and to strengthen the muscles which stabilize them. To work the deep neck flexors.

Starting Position

- Lie on your front, you may place a flat pillow under your forehead to allow you to breathe.
- Your arms are down at your sides, your palms facing your body. Your neck is long. Your legs are together, in parallel with your toes pointing.

Action

1 Breathe in to prepare and lengthen through the spine, and tucking your chin gently in.
2 Breathe out, zip up and hollow and pull your shoulder blades down into your back, lengthening your fingers away from you down towards your feet. The top of your head stays lengthening away from you.
3 Keep looking straight down at the floor. Do not tip your head back. Squeeze your inner thighs together but keep your feet on the floor.

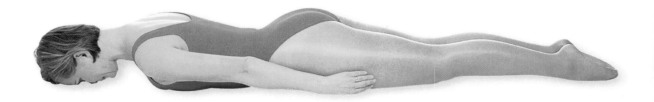

4 Breathe in and feel the length of the body from the tips of your toes to the top of your head.

5 Breathe out, still zipping and hollowing, and release.

Moving on . . .

When you have discovered the wonderful muscles that engage the shoulder blades down into the back, you may add lifting the upper body gently from the floor.

Action

1 Breathe in to prepare and lengthen through the spine, tucking your chin in gently.

2 Breathe out, zip up and hollow and pull your shoulder blades down into your back, lengthening your fingers away from you down towards your feet. The top of your head stays lengthening away from you. Using the mid-back muscles, slowly raise the upper body from the floor. Keep looking straight down. Do not tip your head back. Squeeze your inner thighs together but keep the feet on the floor.

3 Breathe in and feel the length of the body from the tips of your toes to the top of your head.

4 Breathe out, still zipped and hollowed, and slowly lower.

Watchpoints

- Keep hollowing the lower abdominals.
- Do not strain the neck, it should feel released as your shoulders engage down into your back. Think of a swan's neck growing out between its wings.
- Remember to keep your feet on the floor.
- Please stop if you feel at all uncomfortable in the low back. This exercise can also be done with the feet hip-width apart and the thigh and buttock muscles relaxed.

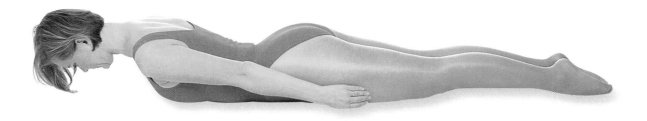

The Big Squeeze

Aim

To work the muscles of the lower abdomen, pelvic floor, the buttocks and the inner thighs, keeping the upper body relaxed.

Starting Position

- Lie on your front. Place a small cushion between the tops of your thighs.
- Rest your forehead on your folded hands, open and relax the shoulders.
- Have your toes together and your heels apart.

Action

1 Breathe in wide and full to prepare and lengthen through the spine.
2 Breathe out, zip up and hollow the lower abdominals to the spine as if there is a fragile egg under the stomach and you do not wish to crush it. Tighten the buttocks, squeeze the inner thighs and the cushion and bring the heels together! Hold for a count of five.

Keep breathing normally and check continually that you are only working from the waist down. Then release. Keep your feet on the floor.
3 Repeat the Big Squeeze five times.

Watchpoints

- Keep your neck and jaw relaxed as you squeeze.
- Feel the full length of your body from the top of your head to the tips of your toes.

Moving on . . .

Try engaging the muscles in this order:
- pelvic floor
- lower abdominals
- buttocks
- inner thighs
- then release in reverse order . . . fun!

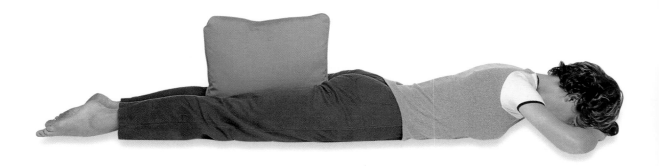

Rest Position

Aim

To lengthen and stretch out your sacral, lumbar, middle and upper spine. To stretch your inner thighs (adductors). To learn control of your breathing in a relaxed position, to sense the filling and emptying of the lungs. To make maximum use of the lungs, taking the breath into the back.

Avoid the Rest Position if you have knee problems as you may compress the joint.

Action

1 Usually this exercise follows one in which you have been lying prone (on your front).
2 Come up onto all fours, bring your feet together, your knees stay apart.
3 Keeping the head and hands still, slowly move back and down towards your buttocks and come to sit on your feet – not between them – the back should be rounded.
4 Rest and relax into this position, leave the arms extended to give you a maximum stretch. Feel the expansion of the back of your ribcage as you breathe deeply into it.
6 The further apart the knees are the more of a stretch you will feel in your inner thighs.
7 With the knees apart further, you can really think of your chest sinking down into the floor.
8 You may also have the knees together which will stretch out the lumbar spine. We do not recommend this version for anyone with back injuries.
9 Take ten breaths in this position.

To come out of the Rest Position

As you breathe out, zip up and hollow and slowly unfurl. Think of dropping your tailbone down and bringing your pubic bone forward. Rebuild your spine vertebra by vertebra until you are upright.

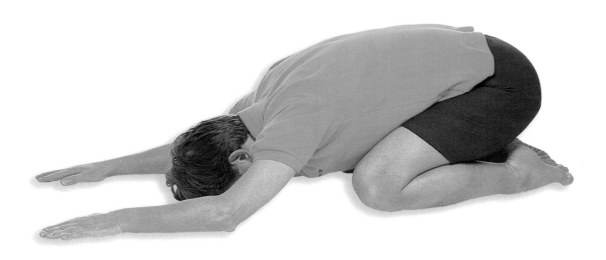

Foot Exercises

Aim

The aim of the following exercises is to work the arches and joints of the foot, promoting mobility and strength.

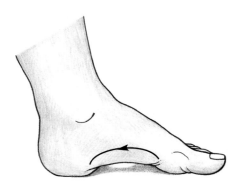

Working the Arches

Starting Position

- You may either sit or stand for this exercise, as long as your body is balanced and comfortable and your feet can remain flat on the floor in parallel.

Action

1 Keeping the toes long and not allowing them to scrunch up, draw the base of your toes back towards the heels thus increasing the arches. Release.
2 Repeat ten times.

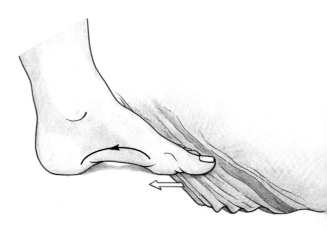

Watchpoints

- Do not simply screw the toes up, the action is in the arches of the feet, not the toes.
- Check that your feet remain evenly planted on the floor and do not roll in or out.

Variation

1 You can lay a scarf or towel out in front of one foot, the edge just resting under your toes.
2 Using the same action as above draw the scarf in towards you.
3 Repeat twice with each foot.

The Mexican Wave

A great party trick, although some people have found this quite difficult so we have added a simpler variation!

Starting Position
As above.

Action
1 Try lifting only your big toes first, keeping the rest down on the floor and then try keeping the big toes down and lifting the other toes.
2 Repeat ten times making sure that your feet do not roll in or out.

The Full Mexican Wave

Action
1 Now try separating your toes and lifting them off the floor one at a time like a Mexican Wave.
2 Then place them back down in sequence, starting with the little toe and spacing them as wide as possible.
3 Repeat five times. You may need to cheat a little to begin with and use your hands to help isolate the toes and move them individually.

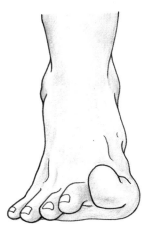
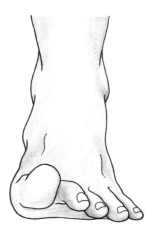
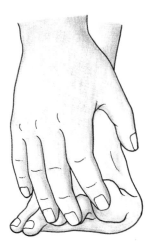

Pointing and Flexing the Feet

Throughout this book we often ask you to either point or flex your feet. It is important that you do this correctly to maintain the right balance in the foot and calf muscles.

Pointing the Feet

Starting Position
- You can practise this sitting or lying in the Relaxation Position with one leg bent and gently extended, held behind the knee.

Action
1 Try softly pointing the foot away from your face, keeping it in a line with the ankle, knee and hip joint.
2 A common mistake is to over-point, which would make the foot 'sickle' inwards. Keep the foot long and make sure that the toes do not curl.
3 Repeat ten times with each foot.

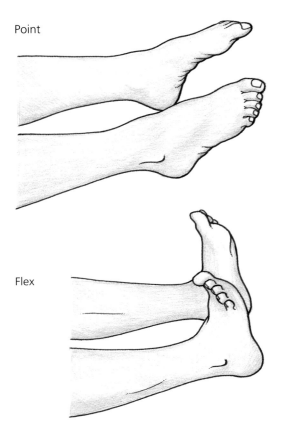

Point

Flex

Flexing the Feet

Action
1 Now try gently flexing the foot, pushing the heel away from your face. The toes will come towards your face but again they should not curl over. Keep them long with the heel lengthening away.
2 Repeat ten times with each foot.

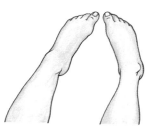
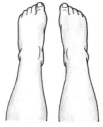

Incorrect point   Correct point

Threading a Needle

Aim

To relax the upper back, especially the muscles round the shoulder girdle.

Starting Position

- Come onto all fours, hands under shoulders, knees under hips, long neck, the head in good alignment with the spine.
- You will be looking straight down at the floor.

Action

1 Breathe in wide and full and transfer your weight onto the right hand.
2 Breathe out, zip up and hollow, lift your left hand and put the back of it on the floor. The elbow is open and relaxed.
3 Slide the left hand along the mat under the right arm, which bends. Keep both shoulders down into the back and relax the head.
4 Breathe in and relax in this position.
5 Breathe out and return to starting point, zipping and hollowing.
6 Repeat three times with each arm.

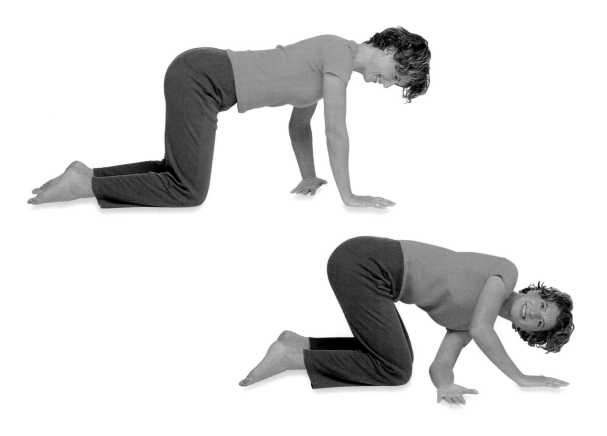

Curl Ups

Aim

To strengthen the abdominals, engaging them in the correct order and with the trunk in perfect alignment. To achieve a flat stomach – well, we all want one!

Please note, you should avoid this exercise if you have neck problems.

Starting Position

- Lie in the Relaxation Position.
- Gently release your neck by slowly rolling the head from side to side.
- Place one hand behind your head, the other hand is on your lower abdomen. This is to check that your stomach does not pop up.
- Your pelvis is in its neutral position.

Action

1 Breathe in wide and full to prepare.
2 Breathe out, zip up and hollow, soften your breastbone, tuck your chin in a little as if holding a ripe peach and curl up, breaking from the breastbone.
3 Your stomach must not pop up. Keep the length and width in the front of the pelvis and the tailbone down on the floor lengthening away. Do not tuck the pelvis or pull on the neck!
4 Breathe in and slowly curl back down.
5 Repeat ten times (change hands after five).

Watchpoints

- Try not to grip round the hips.
- Stay in neutral, tailbone down on the floor and lengthening away. The front of the body keeps its length. a useful image is that there is a strip of sticky tape along the front of the body which should not wrinkle!

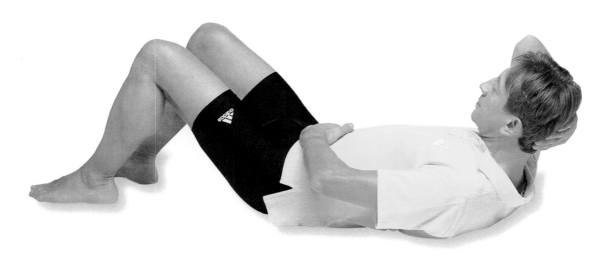

Oblique Curl Ups

Aim

To work the obliques abdominals.

You should avoid this exercise if you have neck problems.

Starting Position

- As for the previous exercise, only place both hands behind your head, the elbows staying open and placed just in front of your ears.

Action

1 Breathe in wide and full to prepare.
2 Breathe out, zip up and hollow and bring your right shoulder across towards your left knee. The elbow stays back, it is the shoulder which moves forward. Your stomach must stay hollow, the pelvis stable.
3 Breathe in and lower.
4 Repeat five times to each side.

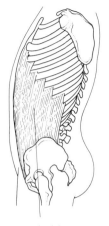 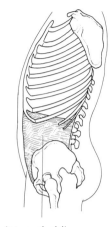

External oblique   Internal oblique

Watchpoints

- As above, making sure that the pelvis stays square and stable.
- Keep the upper body open.
- Keep the neck released.

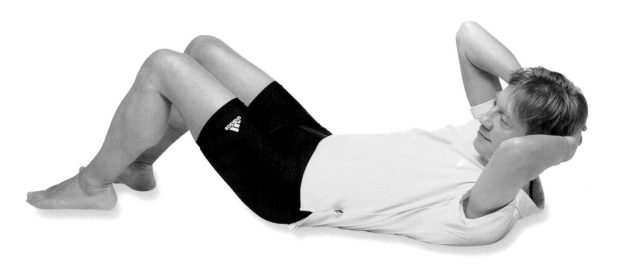

Adductor Stretch

Aim
To stretch the inner thighs, gently, with the pelvis in neutral.

Starting Position
• Lie in the Relaxation Position

Action
1 Breathe in wide and full to prepare.
2 Breathe out, zip up and hollow and bring one knee at a time onto your chest. Breathing normally now, place one hand under each knee and allow the legs to open slowly. This will stretch your inner thighs. Hold this position for two minutes, do not allow your back to arch.
3 After two minutes, still zipping and hollowing, slowly close the legs and return your feet one by one to the floor.

Watchpoint
• Stay in neutral.

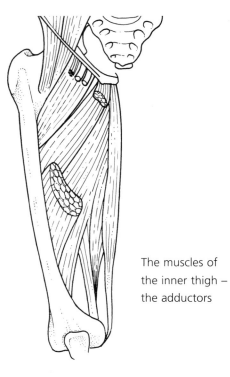

The muscles of the inner thigh – the adductors

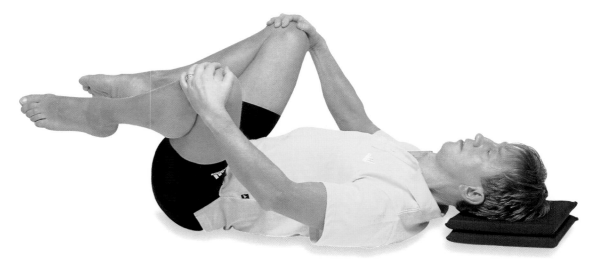

Moving on . . .

Wide Leg Stretch Against a Wall

Aim

A more adventurous stretch for the inner thighs, this is also a lovely position to relax in. With the legs elevated, the 'calf pump' which returns blood to the heart has to work that bit harder, improving your circulation and your lymphatic drainage, thus helping to prevent varicose veins, swelling and to remove toxins.

Starting Position

- Get into the position shown in the photograph – it is easiest to approach the wall sideways and shuffle up as close as you can, then slowly swing the legs up the wall. You must still be comfortable.
- Have a flat pillow to rest your head on.
- Check that you are square onto the wall.
- You may put your hands under your buttocks

if it helps, you should certainly do this if you have back problems. If your hamstrings are tight then come back from the wall a little. Your tailbone must stay down on the floor or you lose neutral.

Note: Come out of this position if you feel any sensations in your legs

Action

1 Now slowly widen your legs until you can feel a stretch on the inner thigh. Allow the legs to bend a little or roll outwards if they wish. The feet should remain level with each other to maintain the correct balance. Try to relax into the stretch working up to about two minutes – there should be no tension anywhere else in the body. You can bring your hands to rest on the abdomen so that the shoulder blades may widen and the elbows release.

2 To come out of the stretch, you may use your hands to help bring the legs together if you wish.

3 Roll slowly onto your side before getting up.

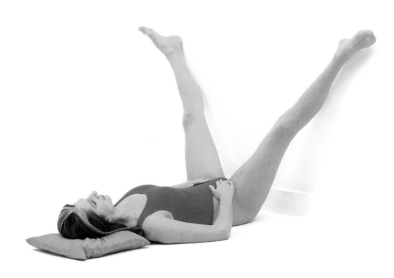

Hamstring Stretch

Aim

To stretch the hamstrings while keeping the torso stable, the back anchored and without creating any tension elsewhere in the body.

The hamstrings are a group of three muscles, so called because in past times farmers would sever the hamstrings of pigs to prevent them from wandering away!

The hamstrings flex and bend the knee. We spend far too much time sitting and, as a result, the hamstrings don't get the natural stretching they need. They can also become tight as they substitute for weak gluteals. So, in addition to gentle hamstring stretches you will also need to strengthen the gluteals through exercises such as The Star on page 114.

If your hamstrings are too short, they will greatly restrict your flexibility and increase the risk of damage to the lumbar spine in everyday forward bending or sport.

Equipment

A long scarf or theraband.

Note: Stop if you feel any strange sensations in your leg.

Starting Position

- Lie in the Relaxation Position.
- You may need a cushion for your head. Bring one knee toward your chest. Hold the scarf from underneath, your palms towards you. Place the scarf over the sole of one foot.

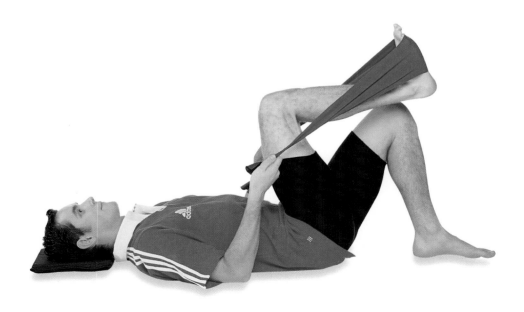

Action

1 Breathe in wide and full to prepare.

2 Breathe out as you zip up and hollow, maintaining neutral 'north to south' pelvic positioning.

3 Slowly straighten the leg into the air. Your tailbone stays down on the floor. Keep your foot relaxed.

4 Breathing normally now, hold the stretch for the count of twenty-thirty seconds.

5 Relax the leg by gently bending it again.

6 Repeat five times to each leg.

To increase the stretch, flex the foot towards your face.

Watchpoints

- Don't allow the pelvis to twist as you straighten the leg – anchoring navel to spine will help you: north to south, east to west.
- Keep your tailbone down as you stretch the leg.
- Check your neck: often the neck shortens and arches back as the hamstrings are stretched. If this happens, place a small flat firm cushion under your head to keep the neck long. Think of softening the neck and breastbone and of opening the elbows. Hold the scarf as for Knee Circles – it will encourage you to keep the shoulder blades down and together.
- Don't strain – ease the leg out, gently stretching it within your limits. Flexing the foot intensifies the stretch.
- Make sure the leg stays in parallel not turning in out.

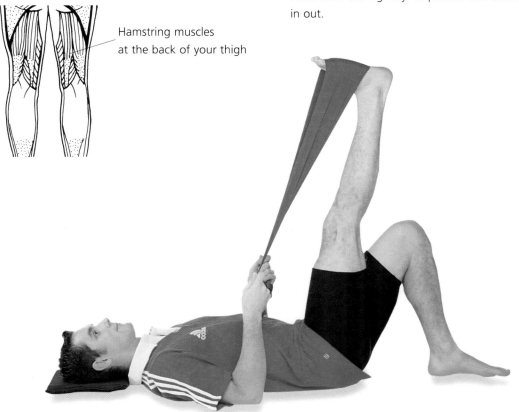

Hamstring muscles at the back of your thigh

Side-Lying Quadriceps and Hip Flexor Stretch

Aim

To stretch out the quadricep muscles which run along the front of the thigh and the hip flexors. To lengthen and iron out the front of the body especially round the front of the hips which can get very tight if you sit all day. To maintain good alignment of the torso by using the waist muscles and shoulder stabilizers.

Please take advice if you have a knee injury. You may need to use a scarf to hook over the foot so that there is less pressure on the knee or you may need to leave this exercise out.

It is crucial that you remain in pelvic and spinal neutral throughout this exercise. Do not allow your back to arch.

Equipment

Scarf and pillow optional.

Starting Position

- Lie on your side, your head resting on your extended arm (you may like a flat pillow between the head and the arm to keep the neck in line).
- Have the knees curled up at a right angle to your body.
- Your back should be in a straight line, but with its natural curve. Line all your bones up on top of each other – foot over foot, knee over knee, hip over hip and shoulder over shoulder.

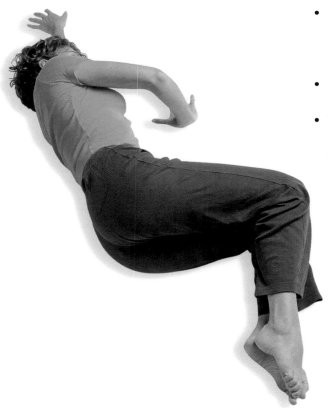

Action

1 Breathe in wide and full to prepare and lengthen through the spine.

2 Breathe out, zip up and hollow and bend the top knee towards you taking hold of the front of the foot if you can reach it (you may need to use a scarf).

3 Breathe in and check that your pelvis is in neutral.

4 Breathe out, still zipping and hollowing and gently take the leg behind you to stretch the front of the thigh. Do not arch the back, keep the tailbone lengthening away from the top of your head.

5 Hold the stretch for about twenty seconds, working the waist the whole time and keeping the length in the trunk.

6 After twenty seconds slowly release by bringing the leg back in front of you, zipping and hollowing throughout.

7 Repeat three times on each side.

Watchpoints

- Keep the waist long.
- Keep the shoulder blades down into the back, and the gap between the arms and the shoulders.
- Do not collapse forward. Keep the upper body open.
- If you cannot reach the foot in the stretch, or the stretch is too great and the knee feels stressed, try using the scarf wrapped over the front of the foot.

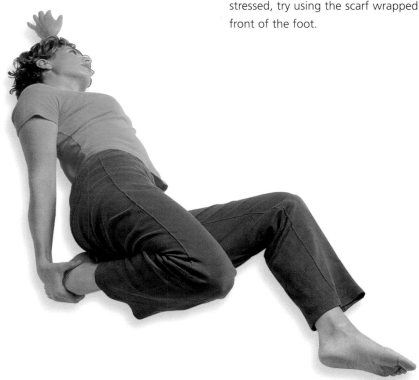

The Pillow Squeeze

Aim

To isolate and work the pelvic floor in conjunction with the deep abdominals, engaging the deep stabilizers. To strengthen the inner thighs. To learn the correct position of the pelvis. To 'open' the lower back.

This is a great exercise if you suffer from the kind of sciatica which is caused by an overactive piriformis muscle.

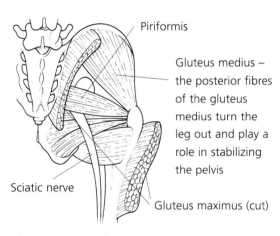

The buttock muscles

Equipment

A plump pillow.

Starting Position

- Lie in the Relaxation Position, but have your feet together flat on the floor.
- Place a cushion between your knees – if you have sciatica, place it at the top between your knees.
- Check that your pelvis is in neutral.

Action

1 Breathe in wide and full to prepare.
2 Breathe out, zip up and hollow and squeeze the cushion between your knees. Keep the pelvis in neutral, the tailbone down on the floor, lengthening away. Try not to grip round the hips.
3 Continue to breathe normally, squeezing and working the pelvic floor and deep abdominals, for a count of up to ten. Then release.
4 Repeat five times.

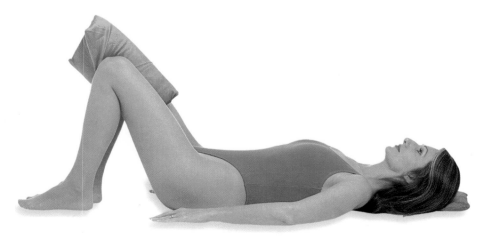

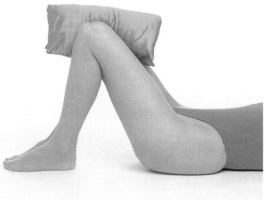

Correct

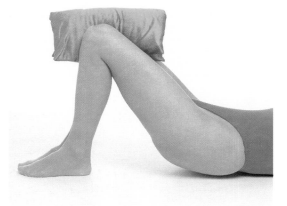

Incorrect: the pelvis has tilted

Watchpoints

- Do not hold your breath, keep breathing.
- Keep your neck released and your jaw soft. You do not need to use your neck to work the pelvic floor!
- The most common mistake made doing this exercise is to lift the tailbone and tuck the pelvis. Think of keeping the length in the front of the pelvis, do not curl or shorten it.

Another good way to check if you are tilting is to place your hand under your waist. Do the exercise wrongly initially, tucking the pelvis and feel the pressure on your hand, you are pushing into the spine. Now try to do the exercise with no pressure on the hand – you have stayed in neutral.

Up and Down with a Tennis Ball

Aim

To learn good alignment of the feet, ankles, knees and hips. To strengthen the large muscle at the front of the thigh (the quadriceps), to stretch the Achilles tendon and calves. To work the stabilizing muscles of the knee, especially vastus medialis.

Starting Position

- Stand sideways on to a wall, and place the tennis ball between your ankles, just below your inside ankle bone.
- You may if you like place another tennis ball or a small cushion between the thighs just above the knees.
- Remind yourself of all the directions given in the last exercise for standing well (page 56).
- Hold onto the wall.

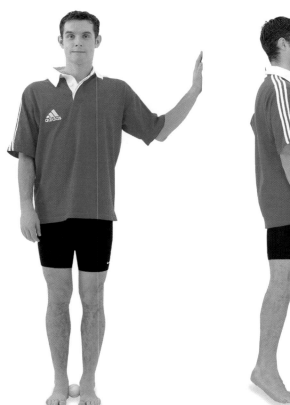
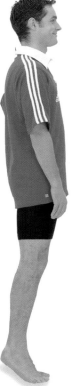
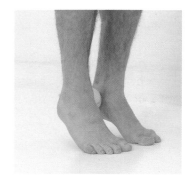

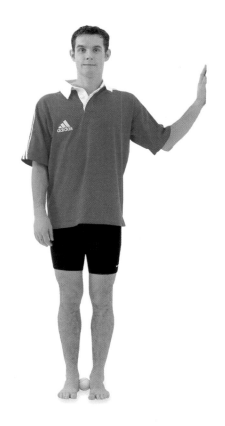
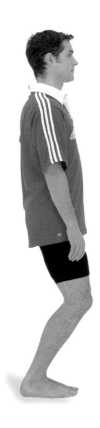

Action

1 Breathe in and lengthen up through the spine – imagine someone is pulling you up from the top of your head, but that there is also a weight on your tailbone, anchoring your spine.

2 Breathe out, zip up and hollow and rise up onto your toes.

3 Breathe in.

4 Breathe out, and slowly lengthen your heels back down on the floor away from the top of your head. Imagine that your head stays up there.

5 When your heels are on the floor, slightly bend your knees directly over your feet, keeping the heels down. Do not allow your bottom to stick out.

6 Repeat ten times.

Watchpoints

- Do not allow your bottom to stick out as you bend the knees.
- Keep the heels on the ground as you bend the knees.
- Keep the weight evenly balanced on the feet.
- Keep lengthening upwards throughout.

A Short Relaxation

Aim

To recognize and release tension from the body. The perfect way to end the day or any of your workout sessions. Ideally you should persuade a friend to read the instructions to you. Otherwise try taping them.

To Relax

- Lie in the Relaxation Position (page 28).
- Allow your whole body to melt down into the floor.
- Allow your body to widen and lengthen.
- Take your awareness down to your feet.
- Soften the balls of the feet, uncurling the toes.
- Soften your ankles.
- Soften your calves.
- Release your knees.
- Release your thighs.
- Allow your hips to open.
- Allow the small of your back to sink into the floor as though you are sinking down into the folds of a hammock.
- Feel the length of your spine.
- Take your awareness down to your hands, stretch your fingers away from your palms, feel the centre of your palms opening.
- Then allow the fingers to curl, the palms to soften.
- Allow your elbows to open.
- The front of your shoulders to soften.
- With each out breath allow your shoulder blades to widen.
- Allow your breastbone to soften.
- Allow your neck to release.
- Check your jaw, it should be loose and free.
- Allow your tongue to widen at its base and rest comfortably at the bottom of your mouth.
- Your lips are softly closed.

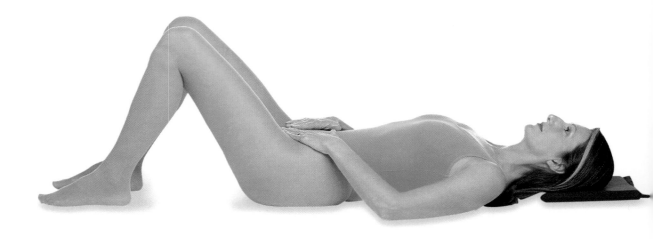

- Your eyes are softly closed.
- Your forehead is wide and smooth and completely free of lines.
- You face feels soft.
- Your body is soft and warm.
- Your spine is released gently down into the floor.
- Observe your breathing but do not interrupt it.
- Simply enjoy its natural rhythm.

To come out of the Relaxation.

1 Very gently allow your head to roll to one side, just allow the weight of the head to take it.
2 Slowly bring it back to the centre and allow it to roll to the other side . . . bring it back to the centre.
3 Then wriggle your fingers . . . and then your toes.
4 Very slowly roll onto one side and rest there for a few minutes before slowly getting up.

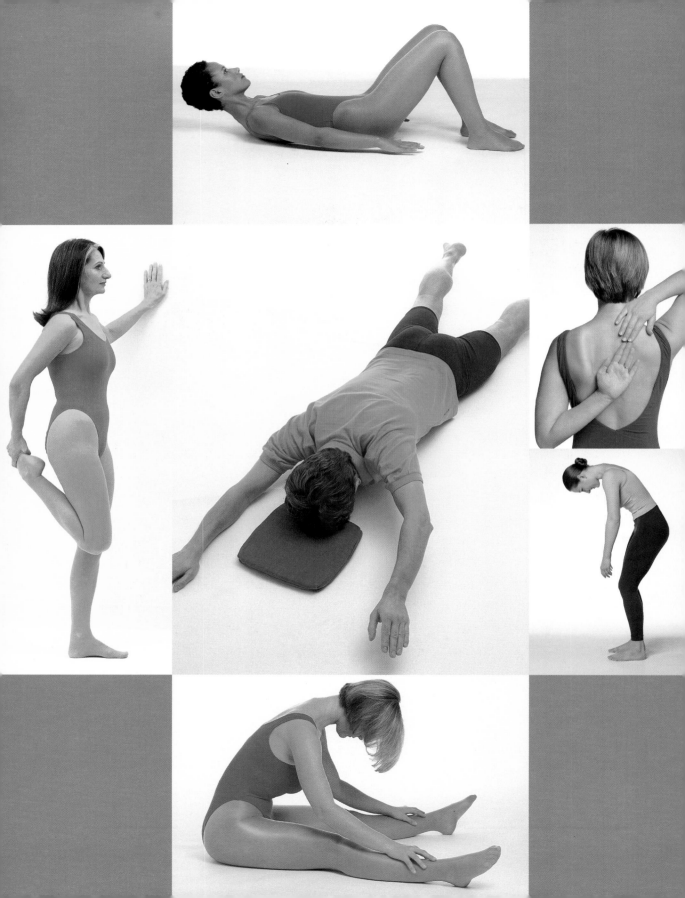

The
Intermediate
Programme

The exercises in the Beginner's Programme have been designed to help you find your true alignment, to isolate and engage the deep stabilizing muscles of the pelvis and spine and to locate and use the stabilizing muscles of the shoulder blades. In addition, you should have a sense of breathing wide and full into the lower ribcage and of being able to move the spine segment by segment safely. Once these skills are mastered, you should have some idea of the girdle of strength round the centre of your body. With this natural corset in place the superficial muscles will be able to release. They, of course, will have also been lengthened by the gentle stretches.

When you are ready, you may begin the Intermediate Programme, which builds on your existing skills. Of course, any of the beginner's exercises may also be included in your intermediate workouts.

Roll Downs (Free Standing)

Aim

To release tension in the spine, the shoulders and the upper body. To mobilize the spine, creating flexibility and strength and achieving segmental control. To teach correct use of the stabilizing abdominal muscles when bending.

A core exercise in any Pilates programme, it can be used as a warm up or a wind down. It combines stabilizing work with the wonderful wheeling motion of the spine. As you roll back up think of rebuilding the spinal column, stacking each vertebra on top of each other to lengthen out the spine.

Please take advice if you have a back problem, especially if disc related.

Starting Position

- Stand with your feet hip-width apart and in parallel, your weight evenly balanced on both feet. Check that you are not rolling your feet in or out. Soften your knees.
- Find your neutral pelvis position but keep the tailbone lengthening down.

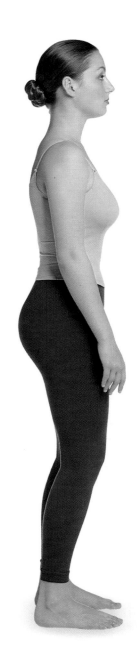

Action

1 Breathe in to prepare and lengthen up through the spine, release the head and neck.

2 Breathe out, zip up and hollow, drop your chin onto your chest and allow the weight of your head to make you roll forward slowly, head released, arms hanging, centre strong, knees soft.

3 Breathe in as you hang, really letting your head and arms hang.

4 Breathe out, firmly zipped and hollowed, as you drop your tailbone down. Directing your pubic bone forward, rotate your pelvis backwards as you slowly come up to standing tall, rolling through the spine bone by bone.

5 Repeat six times.

Watchpoints

- You may like to take an extra breath during the exercise. This is fine but please try to breathe out as you move the spine.

- Make sure that you go down centrally and do not sway over to one side. When you are down, check where your hands are in relation to your feet.

- Do not roll the feet in or out. Keep the weight evenly balanced and try not to lean forward onto the front of your feet or backward onto the heels.

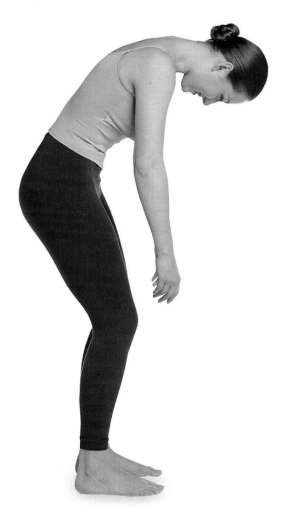

Standing on One Leg

Aim

To learn to balance from within. To work the muscles of the ankles and feet. To work each leg individually. To learn how to achieve pelvic stability, working the deep posterior fibres of gluteus medius.

We all tend to favour one leg which can, as a result, grow stronger than its partner. This can have repercussions throughout the body. Exercises which require you to stand on one leg can help to strengthen the weaker leg. They also work on the gluteus medius, which if weak can cause the opposite quadratus lumborum to become too strong!

It is very useful to do this exercise in front of a mirror so that you can make sure your pelvis stays level. If you find yourself wobbling too much, practise by holding onto the back of a chair.

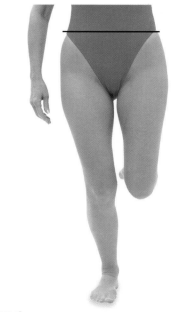

Correct

Starting Position

- Stand in a balanced way, reminding yourself of all the directions given on page 56.

Action

1 Breathe in and lengthen up through the spine.
2 Breathe out, zip up and hollow and take the weight onto one leg keeping the pelvis completely level and without tipping to one side. Lift the other leg a little way off the floor. Keep lengthening up, long waist on both sides.
3 Find your balance and breathe normally for a few breaths before returning the foot to the floor.
4 Repeat five times on each leg.

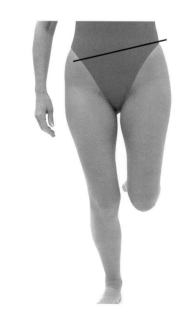

Incorrect

Variation One

This variation demonstrates clearly how much we rely on our visual sense to stay balanced. Without the visual messages to the brain, it has to rely on all the other senses.

Try the above but this time try closing your eyes!

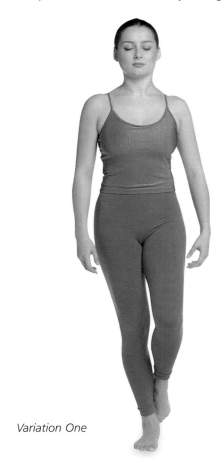

Variation One

Watchpoints
- Try not to sink into the hip of the leg you are standing on.
- Keep lengthening your waist on both sides.
- Do not shift your weight to one side, stay centred.
- The pelvis must stay level.

Variation Two

Follow the instructions above, but this time slide the leg in front of you along the floor, in parallel, then turn the leg out from the hip keeping the pelvis level and still. Make sure that the action originates from the hip and not the knee. Think of the whole leg spiralling out from the hip. Bring the leg back into parallel and slide it back. Repeat five times to each side.

Watchpoints
- Remember how you turned the leg out in Pelvic Stability (page 38) .
- The pelvis stays stable and square.

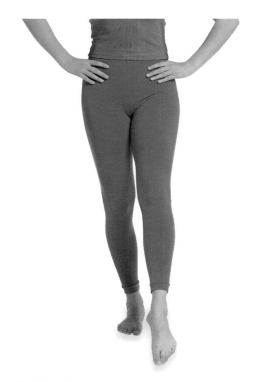

Variation Two

The Corkscrew

Aim

To learn the correct placement and mechanics of the shoulders.

Why is it called the corkscrew? Imagine the type of corkscrew where as the arms are brought down the cork pops up – this is like your head coming up as your arms descend.

Starting Position

• Stand correctly (page 56), weight evenly balanced, spine lengthened, navel to spine.

Action

1 Breathe in to prepare and lengthen up through the spine.

2 Breathe out, zip up and hollow – stay zipped and hollowed now throughout the exercise – and allow your arms to float upwards. Keep the upper shoulders relaxed, think of dropping the shoulder blades down into your back as the arms rise. Clasp your hands lightly behind your head.

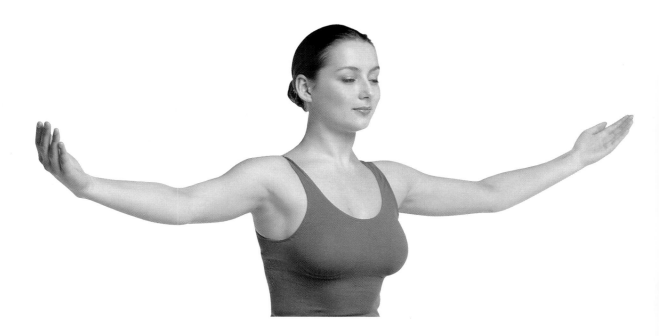

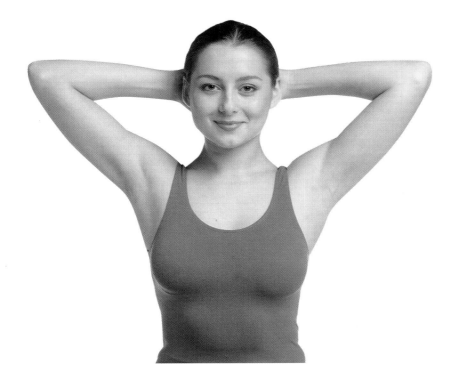

3 Breathe in as you shrug your shoulders up to your ears.

4 Breathe out as you drop them down.

5 Breathe in as you gently bring your elbows back a little. Your shoulder blades will come together. You should be able to still see your elbows.

6 Breathe out as you release your hands and bring them slowly down to your side, opening them wide and engaging the muscles beneath your shoulder blades. As you do this allow the head, neck and spine to lengthen up as the arms come down. Think of a corkscrew.

7 Repeat five times.

Watchpoints

- Remember not to arch the back as you bring your elbows back.
- As you bring the arms up, remember to keep the shoulder blades down for as long as possible by using the muscles below them.

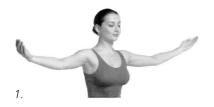

1.

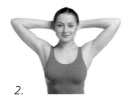

2.

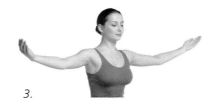

3.

Spine Curls with Pillow

Aim

To learn how to wheel the spine, vertebra by vertebra, achieving synchronous segmental control, using the stabilizing muscles. To work the adductors!

The ability to wheel the spine is an important aspect of the Body Control Pilates programme. Too many of us tend to become locked in one area of the spine.

Equipment

A plump pillow.

Starting Position

• Lie in the Relaxation Position, checking that your feet are in parallel, slightly apart and about 30 centimetres from your buttocks.
• Place the pillow between your knees.

• Your arms are relaxed down by your side, palms down.
• When you are very comfortable with this exercise, you may take your arms above your head, shoulder-width apart.

Action

1 Breathe in to prepare.
2 Breathe out, zip up and hollow, squeeze the cushion between the knees and curl the tailbone off the floor just a little.
3 Breathe in and breathe out, zip up and hollow and slowly curl back down lengthening out the spine.
4 Breathe out, zip up and hollow and peel a little more of the spine off the floor.
5 Breathe in and then breathe out as you place the spine back down, bone by bone.

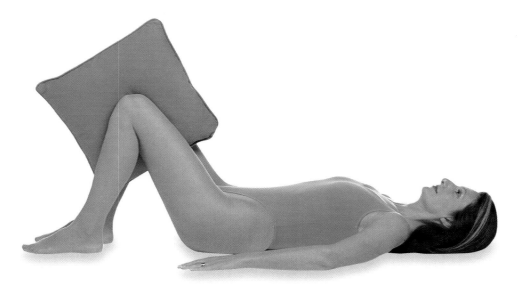

Starting position

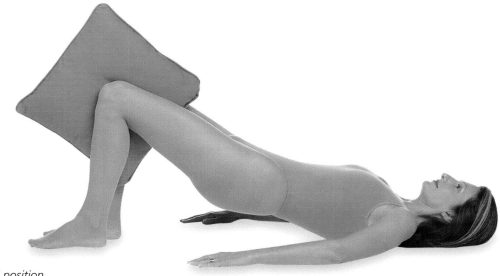

Full position

6 Continue to curl more of the spine off the floor each time you go up on the exhalation. Inhale while you are raised and then exhale as you wheel the spine, vertebra by vertebra, back down to the floor. Aim to lengthen the spine as you wheel back down. The deep abdominals and pelvic floor stay engaged throughout and you keep squeezing the cushion.

7 Finish with a Hip Flexor Stretch (page 47).

Watchpoints

- You must not arch the back. Keep in your mind the image of a whippet who has just been scolded, his tail (your tailbone) curled between his legs!
- Keep the weight even on both feet and try not to let the feet roll in or out.
- Keep your neck long and soft.

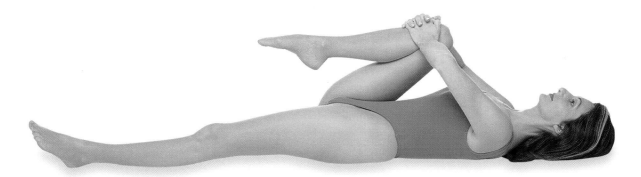

Hip Flexor Stretch

Pelvic Clocks

Aim

To learn pelvic awareness, to work the abdominals. To free the pelvis.

It is believed that this exercise has its origins in the Feldenkrais Method which is a movement therapy.

Starting Position

- Adopt the Relaxation Position and check you are in neutral.

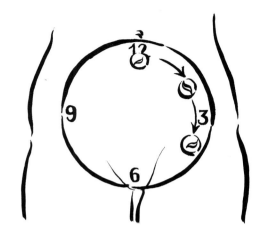

Action

1 Imagine a clock face on your stomach. Your pubic bone is 6 o'clock, your navel 12 o'clock. Visualize a marble sitting in the middle of the clock face. By tilting your pelvis gently, let that marble roll from 6 o'clock to 7 o'clock to 8 o'clock, right round the clock until you reach 6 o'clock again.
2 Try this clockwise and then anti-clockwise!
3 You may notice that your movements are very easy and smooth in some areas while other areas are tight and it is quite an effort to make the marble go round the perimeters. We commonly find that the area between 5 o'clock and 7 o'clock is tighter than the rest.

Once you are more familiar with pelvic clocks in the Relaxation Position, you can also try them:
- Lying on your side in a foetal position (as in the Chalk Circle on page 136).
- On all fours.
- Standing with bent knees, feet hip-width apart.
- Sitting in a chair.

Watchpoints

- Try to keep the movements small and controlled.
- Avoid gripping in the thighs or moving the legs round.

Hip Rolls

Aim

To learn rotation with stability. To work the obliques. To master co-ordination and scapular stabilization.

When you have mastered Side Rolls (page 54) and your abdominals are stronger, you may attempt this more challenging version.

Equipment

A tennis ball.

Starting Position

- Lie on your back, arms out to the side, palms up.
- Your knees should be up towards your chest but in line with your hips. Your thighs will be at right angles to your body. Your feet are softly pointed.
- Place the tennis ball between your knees.

Action

1 Breathe in wide and full to prepare then, as you breathe out, zip up and hollow and slowly lower both legs (a little way at first) towards the floor on your right side while turning your head to the left. Turn the left palm down to remind you to slide the left shoulder blade down your back, keeping it well down on the mat. Also keep the knees in line with each other.

2 Breathe in and breathe out, still zipped up and hollowed and use this strong centre to bring your legs back to the middle. The head also returns to the middle. Your palm turns up.

3 Repeat eight times to each side, going a little further each time but always keeping the opposite shoulder blade down into the back. Think of each part of the back coming off in turn – the buttock, the waist, the lower ribcage – and then returning in reverse order – the back of the ribcage, the waist, the buttock.

Watchpoints

- Keep the opposite shoulder firmly down on the floor.
- Keep the knees in line. Don't go too far unless you can control it.
- Use the abdominals at all times, feel as though you are moving the legs from the stomach.
- Don't allow the weight of your legs to pull you over. Control the movement.
- Do not force the neck the opposite way, allow it to roll comfortably and keep it released and lengthened.

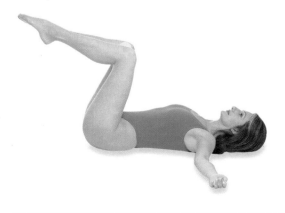
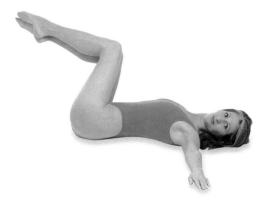

Windmill Arms

Aim

To improve co-ordination, mobilizing the shoulder girdle and improving scapular stabilizing skills.

Starting Position

- Lie in the Relaxation Position, pelvis in neutral, with both arms pointing up to the ceiling, directly above your shoulder joints.
- Long fingers, palms facing towards your feet, elbows soft.

Action

1 Breathe in wide and full to prepare.

2 Breathe out, zip up and hollow and let the right arm move in an arc behind you onto the floor. At the same time the left arm moves towards the hip. This is the same movement as in The Starfish (page 42). The palm of the right hand should face the ceiling, the left hand the floor.

3 Breathe in and slowly move the arms along the floor in opposite directions so that like a

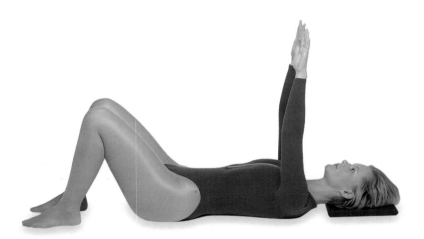

Starting position

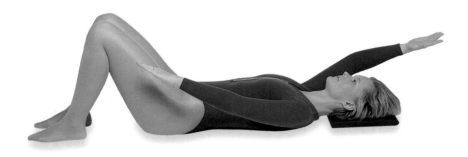

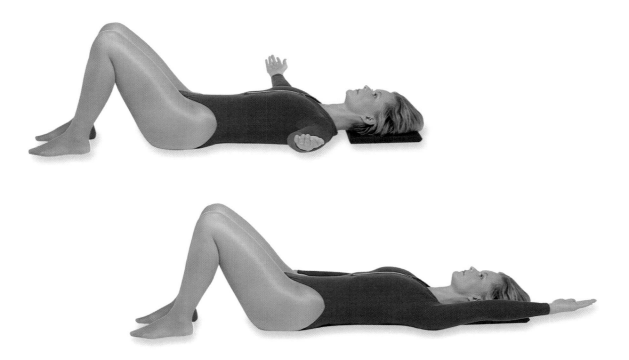

windmill the arms change places You end up with the left hand (palm facing up) behind you and the right hand next to your hip (palm facing down).

4 Breathe out to lift both arms off the mat to return to the starting position.

5 Repeat the same movement five times on each side.

Advanced Version

Reverse the movement after each time – very challenging for the brain!

Watchpoints

- Maintain neutral spine and pelvis throughout.
- Keep the shoulders down and do not force the arms all the way to the mat. Work within your range of movement.

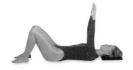
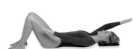
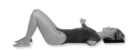
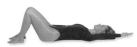

1. Starting position   *2.*   *3.*   *4.*

Curl Ups with Arm Action

Aim

To challenge the abdominals, adding arm movement to improve co-ordination. This exercise is a preparation for the harder abdominal work such as The Hundred where you remain in a curled up position for a considerable length of time.

Remember all the directions already given to you in Abdominal Curl Ups (page 78).

Starting Position

- Lie in the Relaxation Position, checking your neutral pelvis position.
- Clasp both hands behind your head, keeping the elbows open, the shoulder blades down into your back.

Action

1 Breathe in wide and full to prepare.
2 Breathe out, zip up and hollow and, staying zipped up and hollowed throughout, soften your breastbone, tuck your chin in a little and curl up, breaking from the breastbone.
3 Your stomach must not pop up. Keep the length and width in the front of the pelvis and the tailbone down on the floor lengthening away. Do not tuck the pelvis or pull on the neck!
4 Breathe in, still curled up, and take your right hand from behind your head bringing it down alongside your hips, shoulder blades engaged down into your back, reaching down with the fingers.

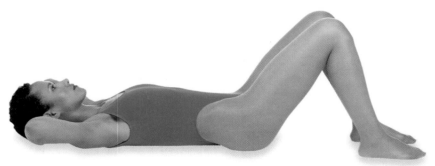

1. Starting position

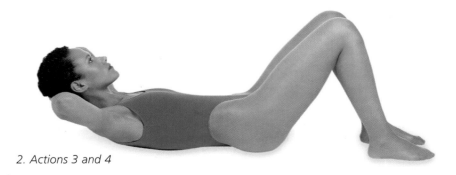

2. Actions 3 and 4

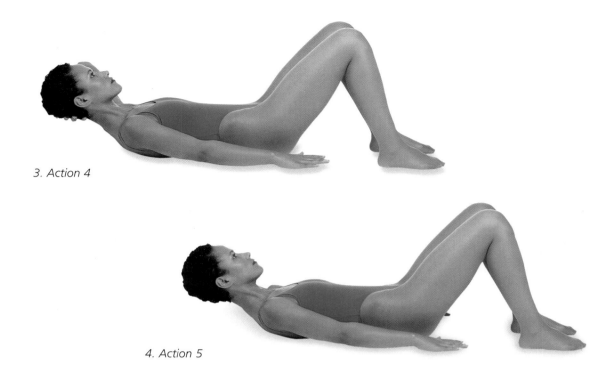

3. Action 4

4. Action 5

5 Breathe out, and repeat the movement with the left hand.

6 Breathe in and bring the right hand back behind your head.

7 Breathe out and bring the left hand back behind your head.

8 Breathe in and slowly lower.

9 Repeat ten times.

Watchpoints

- Keep checking that your pelvis is in neutral and that it doesn't creep up.
- Keep your neck released, if you feel any strain stop.
- Keep zipping and hollowing throughout.
- Really reach through the fingers, shoulder blades connected, and maintain a gap between your ears and your shoulders.

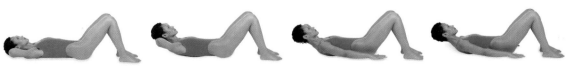

1. Starting position   2.   3.   4.

Single Leg Stretch (Levels One and Two)

Aim
This is a classical Pilates exercise which is best taught in simple stages. It challenges both the abdominals and your co-ordination. In fact it combines *all* the Eight Principles.

Level One

Starting Position
- Lie in the Relaxation Position (page 28), pelvis neutral.

Action
1 Breathe in wide and full to prepare.

2 Breathe out, zip up and hollow and fold one knee at a time up onto your chest.

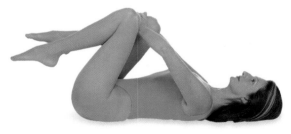

3 Breathe in and with both hands take hold of your right leg under the thigh. Keep your elbows open and your breastbone soft. Your shoulder blades stay down into your back. Neck released.

4 Breathe out, zip up and hollow and slowly straighten the left leg straight up into the air. Keep your back anchored into the floor.

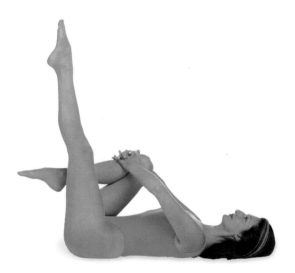

5 Breathe in and bend the left knee back in to your chest. Change hands and hold your left thigh.

6 Repeat ten times with each leg. Do not allow the leg to fall away from you, your back must stay anchored to the floor. When this becomes easy – and only when – you may try the more advanced level two version.

Level Two

This has to be the best abdominal exercise there is!

Starting Position
- Lie in the Relaxation Position.

Action
1 Breathe in to prepare.
2 Breathe out, zip up and hollow and fold your knees up onto your chest one at a time. The toes just touching – but not the heels. Keep your feet softly pointed. Place your hands on the outside of your calves.
3 Breathe in, check that your elbows are open to enable the chest to expand fully. Your shoulder blades are down into your back.
4 Breathe out, zip up and hollow, soften your breastbone and curl the upper body off the floor.

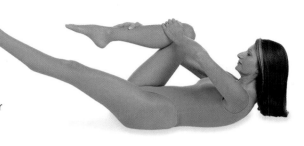

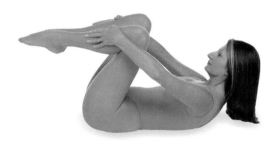

5 Breathe in and place the right hand on the outside of the right ankle, the left hand on the inside of the right knee.
6 Breathe out and, zipping and hollowing, slowly stretch your left leg away in parallel, so that it is at an angle of 45° to the floor. The toes are softly pointed.

7 Breathe in wide and full, as you begin to bend the leg back onto your chest, bringing it back into your shoulder.
8 Change the hands. Your left hand is on the outside of your left ankle, your right hand on the inside of your left knee.
9 Breathe out and, still zipping and hollowing, stretch the right leg away in parallel. Do not take it too close to the floor.
10 Breathe in as the leg returns.
11 Repeat ten stretches on each leg, making sure that you have a strong centre throughout, that your shoulder blades stay down into your back and that your elbows are open.

Watchpoints
- Keep zipping and hollowing throughout and do not allow the back to arch, the pelvis stays neutral.
- Keep your neck released and the upper body open, shoulder blades down.
- Make sure that you keep the length on both sides of your waist, do not allow one side to shorten.

Simple Double Leg Stretch

Aim

To strengthen the abdominals and the deep neck flexors. To co-ordinate breathing and movement. To increase stamina. To strengthen the leg muscles.

A classical Pilates exercise which we have broken down so that you can progress safely and comfortably. The Advanced Version is on page 154. There is also another version in The Series of Five on page 174.

Please take advice if you have neck problems.

Starting Position

- Lie with your knees bent towards your chest.
- Clasp your hands lightly behind your head. Your elbows are open, in a line which passes just in front of your ears. You should be able to see them!

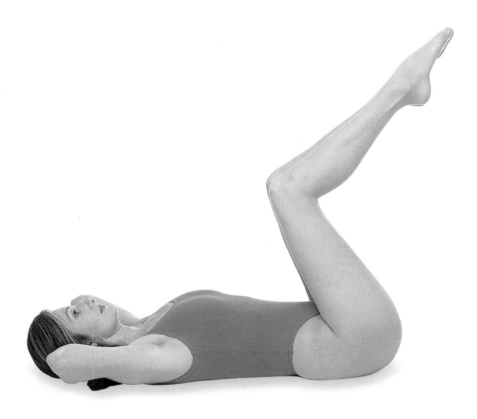

Action

1 Breathe in to prepare.

2 Breathe out, zip up and hollow and slowly curl the head up from the floor, breaking from the breastbone, and keeping the neck soft and long and the chin gently tucked in. As you do so, straighten your legs *as much as is comfortable for you*. The toes are softly pointed. Do not allow them to fall away from you, keep your back anchored into the floor.

3 Breathe in.

4 Breathe out, still zipped up and hollowed and slowly lower your head to the floor, bending your knees onto your chest.

Watchpoints

• Do not pull on the neck, the hands are only there to support the weight of your head.

• Keep a sense of openness in the upper body – do not close in the elbows or the shoulders.

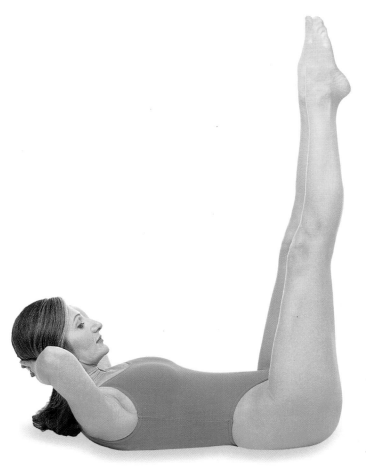

The Diamond Press

Aim

To develop awareness of the scapulae moving on the ribcage. To work the muscles which stabilize the shoulder blades, especially the lower trapezius. To work the deep neck flexors. To encourage lengthening while extending the back.

A subtle exercise which has dramatic results. It really does help to reverse the effects of being hunched over all day. You can feel the tension in your neck release as the stabilizing muscles work.

Starting Position

- Lie on your front with your feet hip-width apart and parallel.
- Create a diamond shape with your arms by placing your fingertips together just above your forehead. Your elbows are open, your shoulder blades relaxed.

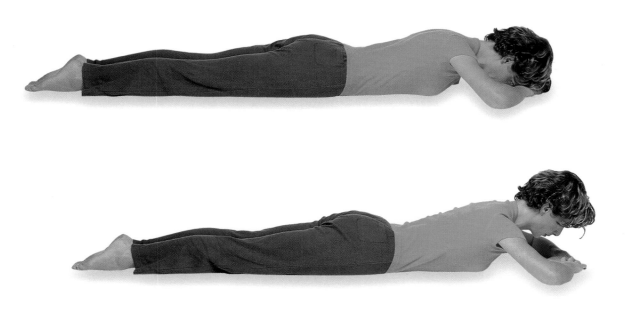

Action

1 Breathe in and lengthen through the spine.

2 Breathe out, zip up and hollow and pull the shoulder blades down into the back of your waist. Gently tuck your chin in to lengthen the back of your neck and lift your head 3 or 4 centimetres off the floor. Stay looking down at the floor, the back of the neck long. Imagine a cord pulling you from the top of your head. Really make the connection down into the small of your back – you have to push a little on the elbows, but think of them connecting with your waist as well.

3 Breathe in and hold the position. Keep the lower stomach lifted, the ribs stay on the floor.

4 Breathe out, still zipped and hollowed and slowly lower back down. Keep lengthening through the spine.

5 Repeat five times.

Watchpoints

• Keep the lower abdominals drawing back to the spine.

• Make sure that you keep looking down at the floor – if you lift your head up you will shorten the back of the neck.

• Keep lengthening from the top of your head to your toes.

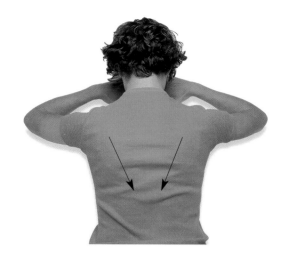

Moving On

When you are comfortable with this movement, add an extra breath so that you hold the position a little longer.

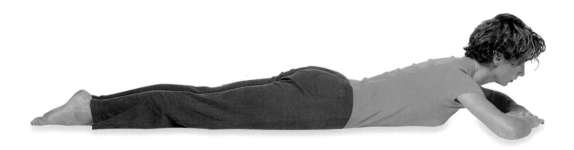

Incorrect

Single Heel Kicks

Aim

To improve co-ordination. To learn how to extend the back safely with stability. To stretch the quadriceps gently and to strengthen the hamstrings. To mobilize and articulate the ankle joints.

This exercise can be carried out either in a sphinx position (photo one) with the upper back extended or with the head down, resting on folded hands (photo two). You should be comfortable with the Diamond Press and Dart exercises before you attempt to extend the back further.

Please take advice if you have a back or knee injury.

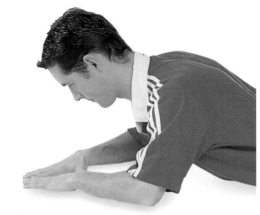

1. Sphinx position

Starting Position

- Lie on your front.
- If you are coming up into a sphinx position as in photo one – place the hands on the floor just creating a diamond shape as for The Diamond Press page 110.
- Zipping and hollowing, push down onto the forearm to raise the upper body off the floor. The elbows stay down. Make sure that your neck remains long, the shoulders well away from the ears and the breastbone. Your pelvis and pubic bone remain on the floor, navel lifted to the spine throughout the exercise. You should feel comfortable in this position – if you feel any pinching in your back, come down to the alternative position.
- In the alternative position, rest your forehead on your folded hands. Make sure that your upper back remains open and relaxed (photo two).

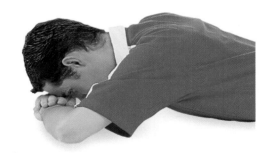

2. Folded hands

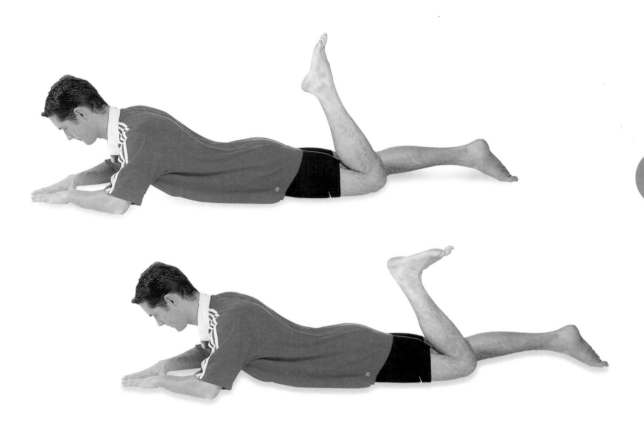

Action

1 With the legs slightly apart, zip up and hollow and kick the right foot into the buttocks, keeping the foot pointed. Release the leg slightly then flex the foot and kick again.
2 Repeat with the other foot.
3 Breathe normally throughout the exercise.
4 Repeat eight times with each leg.

Watchpoints

- If you are in the sphinx position do not allow yourself to sink down, keep lengthening, zipping and hollowing.
- In either position, make sure that both hips stay in balanced contact with the floor.

The Star

Aim

To learn how to work from a strong stable centre. To work the deep gluteal muscles and the upper back muscles. To learn how to extend the leg safely.

If you are uncomfortable lying on your stomach, place a small, flat cushion under your abdomen to tilt the pelvis and start gently. If you have a history of sciatica leave the legs in parallel.

We have given you two stages to this exercise.

Stage One

Starting Position

- Lie on your front have your feet hip-width apart, turned out from the hips (see note above).
- Rest your forehead on your folded arms.

Action

1 Breathe in to prepare and lengthen through the spine.
2 Breathe out, zip up and hollow. Lengthen, then raise the left leg lifting it no more than 5 centimetres off the ground. Lengthen away from a strong centre. Do not twist in the pelvis, both hip bones stay on the floor. Try to keep your shoulders relaxed and a sense of width in your upper body.
3 Breathe in and relax.
4 Repeat five times with each leg.

Watchpoints

- Keep the lower abdominals supporting your lower back.
- Think of creating space round the hip joint as you lengthen the leg away.
- Be careful to keep both hip bones on the floor – you are only lifting the leg.
- Don't let the pelvis roll or twist, keep it square.
- Keep your neck long and relaxed, the head stays down on the floor throughout the exercise.
- Everyone lifts the legs too high, so aim to lift just a few centimetres.

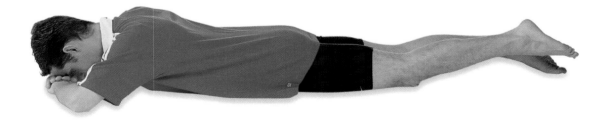

Stage Two: The Full Star

Starting Position

- Take your arms out just wider than shoulder width so that you look like a star, but remember to leave your shoulder blades set down in your back.
- You may like to place a small, very flat, pillow or folded towel under your forehead. The cushion should not alter the angle of your neck.

Action

1 Breathe in to prepare and lengthen through the spine.
2 Breathe out, zip up and hollow and lengthen. Then raise the opposite arm and leg no more than 5 centimetres off the ground. Lengthen away from a strong centre. Do not twist in the pelvis, both hip joints stay on the floor. Try to keep a sense of width in your upper body.
3 Breathe in and relax.
4 Repeat with opposite side.
5 Repeat five times each side.
6 When you have finished The Star come onto all fours and back into the Rest Position (page 73), do not do this if you have a knee problem.

Watchpoints

- As for Stage One.
- Do not overreach or overlift the arms. Keep the elbows slightly bent and keep them wide.
- Keep your neck long and relaxed, the head stays down on the floor throughout the exercise.
- Do not overreach with the arms. Keep the elbows slightly bent and keep them wise.

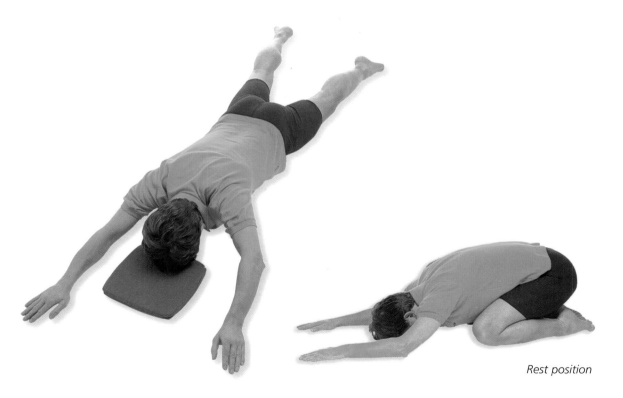

Rest position

Lying Side Stretch

Aim

To strengthen muscles of the waist while keeping good alignment. To work the muscles which stabilize the shoulder blades. To strengthen the muscles which run along the side of the hip and leg.

Starting Position

- Lie on your side, your underneath leg bent, the thigh at an angle of about 70° to the torso, the upper leg in line with the torso.
- Your head should be in line with the spine and the underneath arm stretched out in line with the torso (if this is uncomfortable, stretch the arm out at a right angle to the torso and use a thick head support).
- Line up shoulder over shoulder, hip over hip.
- The working leg should be lined up with the torso and remain straight with the foot flexed.
- The upper arm lengthens along the body, palm resting on top of the thigh.

Action

1 Breathe in wide and full to prepare, the top leg stays straight with the foot on the floor – lengthen away through the heel out of the hip.
2 Breathe out, zip up and hollow and lift the top leg, in parallel, just above hip level. At the same time bend from the waist, reaching with the arm towards the knee, sliding the hand along the leg. Eventually your head comes off the mat, this happens as part of the movement of the torso. Keep your head, neck and spine in good alignment throughout.
3 Breathe in to lower and rest.
4 Repeat up to eight times each side.

Watchpoints

- Keep the top leg in parallel.
- Focus straight ahead and maintain correct alignment of trunk and head.
- Keep a long underneath waistline and an open chest.
- If this exercise strains your neck, rotate the head down towards the floor and keep the back of your neck long.

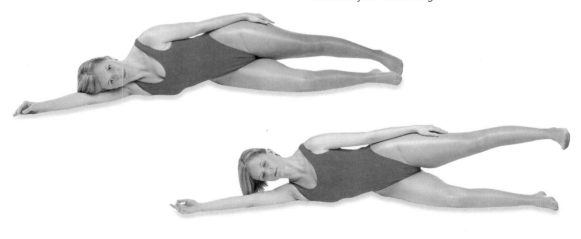

Tricep Stretch

Aim

To stretch the triceps at the back of the upper arm. To open the upper body, enjoying lateral breathing.

Equipment

A scarf or theraband

Starting Position

- Sit or stand with your pelvis in neutral.
- Place one hand on the back of your head, at the top of your spine, the other hand at the base of the spine.
- Keep a sense of openness in the front of your body, but do not allow the back to arch.

Action

1 Breathe in to prepare and lengthen up through the spine.

2 Breathe out, zip up and hollow and start tracing the spine with your fingers until both hands meet. Quite probably they will not be able to meet – please do not force them! If you have your scarf with you, you can hold onto each end to bring the hands closer – but never strain. Do not allow your upper back to arch.

3 Take two deep breaths, keeping your head central and your ribs wide.

4 Breathe out, zip up and hollow and slowly trace down the spine as you take your arms back to the starting position.

5 Repeat three times on each side. It is common for one side to be harder than the other.

Watchpoints

- Do not allow the head to twist or tilt to one side.
- Do not allow the back to arch.

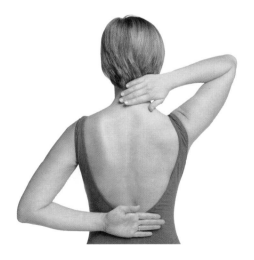
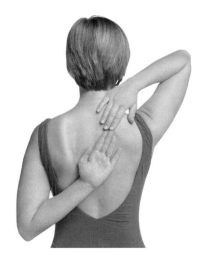

Table Top

Aim

To learn how to keep your centre stabilized while moving the limbs, maintaining neutral and keeping the length in the trunk. To learn balance and control. To learn pelvic stability and to work the deep gluteals.

The key to this exercise is keeping your girdle of strength working, supporting the spine and keeping both sides of the waist long, the pelvis neutral and level. No tension should creep into the upper body.

A complementary exercise would be Standing on one Leg, page 94.

Stage One

Starting Position

- Kneel on all fours, your hands directly beneath your shoulders, your knees beneath your hips. Check that your pelvis is neutral, the natural curve maintained.

Action

1 Breathe in wide and full to prepare as you lengthen the spine from the top of your head to your tailbone.
2 Breathe out, zip up and hollow and slide the left leg away from you, straightening it along the floor. Your back and pelvis stay still.
3 Breathe in and slowly return the leg.
4 Repeat five times with each leg. Keeping the pelvis level and stable. Try to keep the weight transfered through the hands even on both sides.

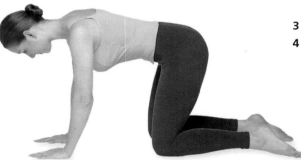

Starting position

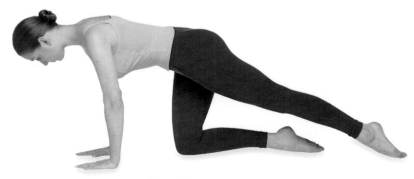

Stage One

Stage Two (Table Top with Sliding Legs)

When you have mastered the above – always keeping your centre stable – you may try the next stage.

Action
Follow steps 1–3 above then:

4 After lengthening the leg along the floor, breathe in and out as you lift the leg slowly to hip height – and no higher! The pelvis must stay absolutely level, do not allow the low back to dip. Again try to keep the weight even on your hands.

Stage Three

Action
When you can lift the leg easily, follow steps 1 to 4 in the previous stage and then:

5 As you lift the leg on the out breath, simultaneously lift and lengthen the opposite arm at shoulder height. Do not overreach. Keep the shoulder blade down and the neck long. The pelvis stays square to the floor. Keep looking at the floor, the top of the head lengthening away from the tailbone.

6 Breathe in and lower the arm and leg.

7 Repeat five times, alternating arms and legs.

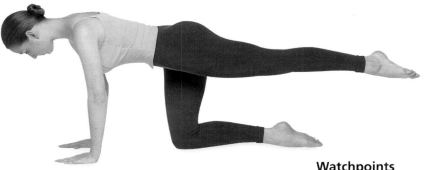

Stage Two

Watchpoints
- Keep the lower abdominals engaged throughout.
- Do not allow the pelvis to tilt to one side.
- Keep looking straight down at the floor – if you raise your head you will shorten the back of your neck.

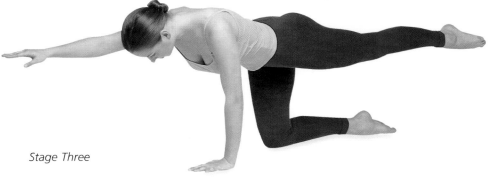

Stage Three

The Hundred (Stages One to Four)

Aim

To learn the breathing pattern of The Hundred, which involves lateral lower ribcage breathing to a set rhythm. To strengthen the pectoral muscles. To master stabilizing the shoulder blades. To strengthen the abdominals.

The Hundred is one of the classical Pilates exercises. It used to be the warm up exercise for mat classes. Well, it certainly warms you up! We have broken the exercise down into manageable bite-sized chunks. When you have mastered one stage, you may proceed to the next. This first stage tackles the breathing pattern, which stimulates the circulatory system, oxygenating the blood.

Please take advice if you have neck, respiratory or heart problems.

Stage One

Breathing Preparation

- Lie in the Relaxation Position. Place your hands on your lower ribcage. Breathe in wide and full into your sides and back for a count of five. Breathe out, zip up and hollow, for a count of five.
- Repeat ten times, staying zipped and hollowed for both the in and the out breaths. If you find the count of five too difficult try the count of three.

Stage Two

Starting Position

- Lie in the Relaxation Position. You may use a firm flat cushion under your head if you wish.
- Zipping and hollowing bend your knees up onto your chest one at a time and in parallel. Your arms are extended alongside your body, palms down, wrists straight.
- Leave your head down on the floor.

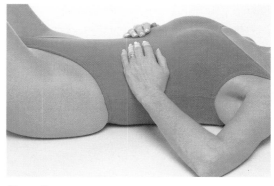

Stage One

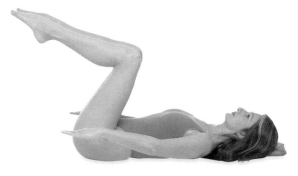

Stage Two

Action

1 Breathing in wide into your sides and back, pump your arms up and down, no more than 15 centimetres off the floor for a count of three or five. The shoulder blades stay down with the fingers lengthening away.

2 Breathe out and pump the arms for a count of three or five.

3 Repeat at least ten times, working up to twenty repetitions, hence 'The Hundred'.

Watchpoints

- Your breathing should be comfortable. Do not over breathe. If you feel light-headed take a break.
- As you beat the arms be aware of any unnecessary tension in your neck, keep the neck released.
- Your shoulder blades should stay down into your back as your arms lengthen away.

Stage Three

Aim

To continue with the breathing training and add abdominal training. To work the deep neck flexors, while keeping the superficial neck muscles released.

Starting Position

- Lie in the Relaxation Position. Bring your knees up onto your chest, one at a time, keeping the legs in parallel. Arms down by your side. Slowly roll your head from side to side to release your neck.

Action

1 Breathe in wide and full to prepare.

2 Breathe out, zip up and hollow and curl the upper body off the floor, remembering

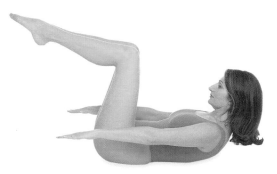

Stage Three

everything you learnt for Curl Ups (page 78): chin gently tucked forward, relaxed jaw, soft breastbone, released neck.

3 Zipped and hollowed, start the breathing and pumping action of the arms which you mastered in stage two. Breathe in laterally for five beats and out for five beats. Keep the shoulder blades down and a large gap between your ears and your shoulders.

4 Repeat twenty times until you reach one hundred, then slowly return the feet to the floor and lower your head.

Watchpoints

- Return to the floor if you feel any strain at all in your neck.
- To prevent strain and engage the deep stabilizers, have your chin gently tucked in but not squashed. Your line of focus should be between your thighs. The back of your neck remains long, the front relaxed.
- You must keep breathing wide into your lower ribcage or you will become breathless. If you do feel breathless, stop at once.
- Keep a sense of width in your upper body. Do not close in your shoulders, keep the upper body open, the breastbone soft. ▷

Stage Four

Please take advice if you have neck, respiratory or heart problems.

Starting Position
- Lie in the Relaxation Position zipping and hollowing.
- Bring your knees up onto your chest, one at a time, keeping the legs in parallel. Arms down by your side, pelvis in neutral.
- Slowly roll your head from side to side to release your neck.

Action
1 Breathe in wide and full to prepare.
2 Breathe out, zip up and hollow and curl the upper body off the floor, remembering everything you learnt for Curl Ups (page 78) – chin tucked gently forward, relaxed jaw, soft breastbone, released neck.

3 Breathe in and then out as, zipped and hollowed, you straighten the legs into the air as much as you are comfortable. Do not allow them to fall away or your back will arch – it must stay anchored to the floor, the pelvis in neutral. Your feet are softly pointed.
4 Zipped and hollowed, start the breathing and pumping action of the arms which you mastered in the last exercise. Breathe in laterally for five beats and out for five beats. Keep the shoulder blades down and a large gap between your ears and your shoulders.
5 Repeat twenty times until you reach 'One Hundred', then slowly bend your knees onto your chest and lower your head.

Watchpoints
- Return to the floor if you feel any strain at all in your neck.
- To prevent strain and to engage the deep stabilizers, have your chin gently tucked in – but not squashed! Your line of focus should be between your thighs. The back of your neck remains long, the front relaxed.
- You must keep breathing wide into your lower ribcage or you will become breathless. If you do feel breathless, stop at once.
- Keep a sense of width in your upper body. Do not close the shoulders in, keep the upper body open, the breastbone soft.

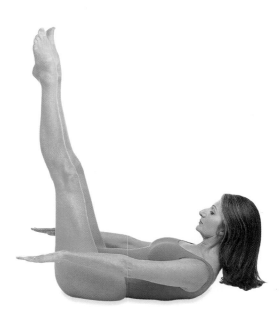

Stage Four

Beach Ball Hamstring Stretch

Aim

To lengthen and stretch the hamstring muscles and the back muscles gently. To reinforce scapular stabilization and lateral breathing.

The hamstrings are mobilizing muscles which have a tendency to take on the role of stabilizing when the body is out of alignment and has no core stability. As a result they can become very tight. If you have in the past found that in spite of continual stretching, they still will not lengthen, then your muscles need balancing.

Please take advice if you have a knee, hip or disc injury.

Starting Position

- Sit with your knees bent and the soles of your feet together. Do not bring the feet too close to your body, you should be comfortable.
- Your pelvis should be square. Straighten one leg out in front of you, in a line with your hip and in parallel (knee cap facing the ceiling). The sole of the foot of your bent leg is resting on the inside of your knee. Your foot is relaxed.
- If you find it easier you may like to sit on a rolled up towel.

Action

1 Breathe in to prepare and lengthen up through the spine.
2 Breathe out, zip up and hollow, lift up out of your hips and gently stretch forward. Do not twist over one leg but stay in the centre.
3 Take twelve breaths in this position, relaxing into the stretch. Breathing wide and full into the lower ribcage and back. Your neck is long, your shoulder blades down into your back, your arms resting in front of you. Keep your weight even on both sitting bones.
4 If you wish, you may take the arm which is on the same side as the bent knee behind you and rest the hand, palm up, facing backwards. The arm on the side of the straight leg rests alongside the leg. This helps keep your shoulders straight (see photo).
5 After twelve breaths, on the next out-breath, zip up and hollow and slowly rebuild the spine vertebra by vertebra.
6 Repeat on the other side.

Watchpoints

- Keep the top of your head lengthening away, your jaw relaxed and your chin gently tucked in.
- Do not lock the knee back, the straight leg stays straight but relaxed.

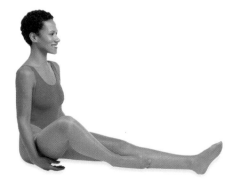
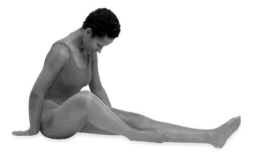

The Spine Stretch

Aim

To stretch the spine and the inner thighs gently. To focus on lateral lower ribcage breathing. To stabilize the trunk.

The wider you place your legs the greater the stretch. This will depend on the flexibility of your hips and the length of your hamstrings. Please do not overstretch.

Starting Position

- Sit on your sitting bones with your legs in front of you. If you like you may sit on a rolled up towel. It will help you to keep your pelvis at the right angle. You could also try sitting with your buttocks up against the wall.
- Now, take your legs a comfortable distance apart but do not force the knees down onto the floor, they may remain a little bent if necessary. Have your toes softly pointed until you are very flexible, you can then have your feet flexed.

Action

1 Breathe in to prepare and lift up out of the hips and lengthen up through the spine. Imagine that there is a pole behind you along your spine, lengthen up along the pole.
2 Breathe out, zip up and hollow and drop your chin forward, gently tucking it in. Then, like a roller blind, curl downwards aiming the top of your head towards the centre of your stomach. Reach forward with your hands.
3 Continue to breathe normally, still zipped and hollowed, inch forwards reaching through the fingers. If you are flexible enough try to press the knees into the floor, lengthening through the heels.
4 After eight breaths, zipped and hollowed still, slowly start to unfurl, re-stacking the vertebra one on top of the other until the spinal column is rebuilt along the length of the imaginary pole. Bring your head up last of all.
5 Repeat three times.

Watchpoints

- Keep your shoulders down into your back, your neck long and released.
- Keep breathing into the back of your ribcage.

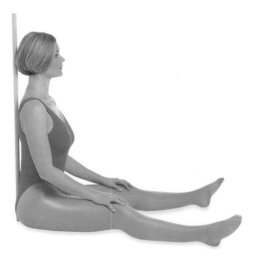

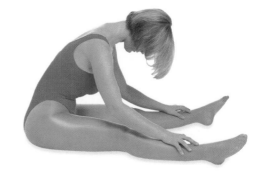

The Arm Weight Series: Working with Arm Weights – Flys

Aim
To open the upper body, teaching correct upper-body use. To tone the chest and upper arm muscles. To work the inner thighs. To increase bone density.

Equipment
Arm weights of up to 2 kilograms – please start with half-kilo weights and gradually increase the weight as you become stronger. Only use two-kilo weights if you are already very strong and want more defin-ition in the arms. If you have no weights use a bag of rice or dried beans instead.

Tennis ball or pillow.

Starting Position
- Lie on your back, knees bent and together. Put the tennis ball between the knees. Feet flat.
- Extend the arms, keeping the natural shape of the arm with the elbows slightly bent, as if you are hugging a large tree trunk

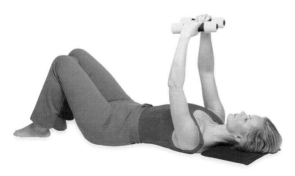

- Throughout the exercise you will be zipping and hollowing, gently squeezing the pillow or tennis ball, pelvis in neutral of course.

- If you can lie on a narrow bench to get the full benefit of opening the chest.

Action
1 Breathe in, as you open the arms directly to the side onto the floor, again keeping the natural shape. The elbows stay slightly bent.
2 Breathe out, as you bring the arms back over your chest to be line with your breastbone.

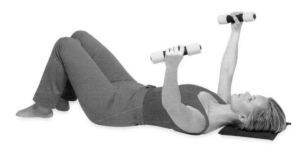

3 Keep squeezing the inner thighs together and hollowing out the lower abdominals.
4 Repeat ten times.

Watchpoints
- Don't unfold the arms, i.e. don't hinge from the elbow – keep the natural curve.
- Take the arms directly to the side, rather than taking the weight behind you.
- Keep hollowing the abdominals – remember north to south, neutral spine.
- Keep squeezing those inner thighs, but don't lift the tailbone – keep it lengthening away.

The Arm Weight Series: Backstroke Swimming

Aim

To learn correct shoulder movement, stabilizing the shoulder blades. To open the shoulder blades. To combat round shoulders. To work the adductors.

A wonderful exercise to counter those hunched positions we all find ourselves in everyday. Enjoy the sensation of opening out.

Equipment

Hand weights of between 0.5 to 1.0 kilogram.
Tennis ball or pillow.

Starting Position

- Lie in the Relaxation Position on a narrow bench if possible. Your feet are together lined up perfectly.
- Place a tennis ball between the knees.
- Holding the hand weights, raise your arms to the ceiling, palms away from your face with your elbows slightly bent. Throughout the exercise you will be zipping and hollowing and gently squeezing the pillow or tennis ball.

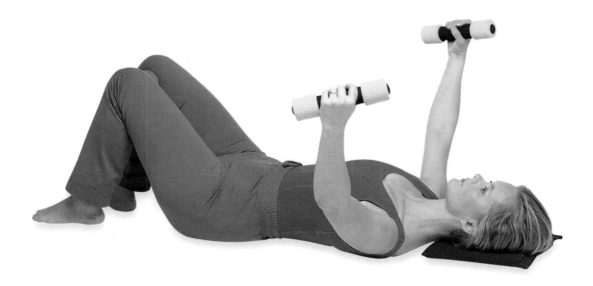

Action

1 Breathe in wide and full to prepare.

2 Breathe out, zip up and hollow, as you take the right arm behind you to the floor, the left hand down to the side of your hip.

3 Breathe in as you bring the arms back up to the starting position.

4 Breathe out as you repeat the movement to the other side.

5 Keep squeezing the inner thighs and hollowing the lower abdominals.

6 Repeat ten times to each side.

Watchpoints

• Neutral pelvis please.

• As you take the arm behind you, keep it outside the line of the shoulder.

• If you are using a bench, keep the arm in line with the body and parallel to your side.

• Keep squeezing the inner thighs together, but don't lift the tailbone.

• Keep a sense of openness in the upper body and keep those shoulder blades engaged down into the back.

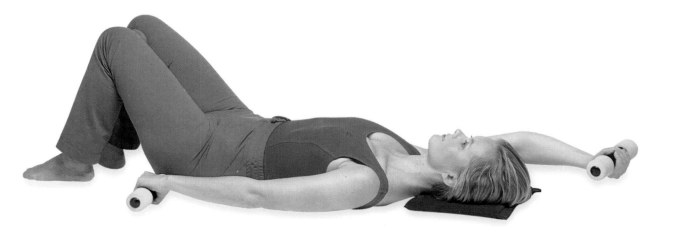

The Arm Weight Series:Triceps

Aim

To strengthen the triceps without compromising the neck. If using a cushion, to strengthen the inner thighs.

There are lots of ways to work the triceps. This one is great because there is no risk of overusing your neck muscles. You will need to take a firm grip on the weight.

Equipment

A weight. You can either buy a long hand-held weight or use a tall can or heavy rolling pin. They should each weigh between 1 to 3.5 kilograms. Obviously start with the lightest weight and work up.

You may also need a cushion or tennis ball.

Starting Position

- Lie with your knees bent, pelvis in neutral.
- If you wish you may place a small cushion or tennis ball between your knees and throughout the exercise you can squeeze the cushion to work the inner thighs.

- Hold the weight at each end, with your palms facing upwards. Your elbows are bent directly over your shoulders, your upper arms are vertical to you.

Action

1 Breathe in to prepare.
2 Breathe out, zip up and hollow and slowly straighten your arms, keeping the elbow quite still. Do not fully straighten the arms, stop just short.
3 Breathe in as you lower.
4 Repeat up to twenty times.

Watchpoints

- Keep that firm grip on the weight.
- Keep your neck released and your shoulder blades down into your back.
- If you are squeezing the cushion between your knees, be sure that you do not tilt the pelvis or grip round the hips – see Pillow Squeeze on page 86.

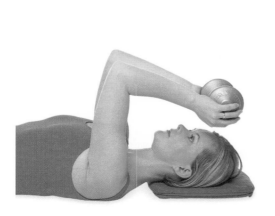
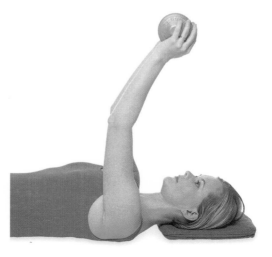

The Arm Weight Series: Biceps

Aim
To strengthen the bicep muscles, while stabilizing the shoulder blades.

Equipment
Hand-held weights, each weighing up to 2.5 kilograms.

Starting Position
- Stand correctly, reminding yourself of all the directions on page 56.
- Hold the weights in your palms facing inwards.

Action
1 Breathe in wide and full to prepare, lengthening up through the spine.
2 Breathe out zip and hollow and raise one arm, keeping the elbow quite still and close into your side, turning the arm so that your palm now faces backwards. Your hand will finish close to your shoulder joint.
3 Breathe in as you return it to your side.
4 Repeat ten times with one arm, and then switch to the other. Work up towards doing a set of three on each side, stay zipped and hollowed throughout.

Watchpoints
- Keep the elbow isolated and still. If you find it keeps moving, put the other weight down and put the hand just inside the elbow to steady it.
- Keep reminding yourself of the correct standing instructions, lengthening up through the spine.
- Keep your shoulder blade down into your back, and your upper body open.
- Do not be tempted to rock forward and back.

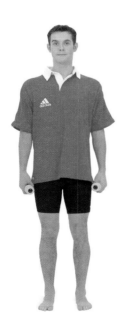 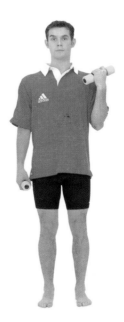

The Leg Weight Series – Abductor Lifts and Twenty Lifts

Aim

This series of exercises is designed to strengthen the outer thigh muscles (abductors) and the gluteals. It also tones the upper leg and controls cellulite.

These two exercises will challenge your pelvic and lumbar stability so you must be stable before you attempt them. Good preparation exercises are the pelvic stability exercises, Standing on One Leg and Table Top with Sliding Legs (pages 94 and 119).

Equipment

Practise these exercises without weights first, until you are totally familiar with them and they cause you no discomfort. You may then strap leg weights of up to 1.5 kilograms onto your ankles. Start with the lightest weight.

Starting Position

- Lie on your left side in a straight line – this is crucial, so, if you like, you can lie up against a wall to check your alignment. Don't lean on the wall!
- Remember neutral please.
- Your left arm is stretched out, your head resting against the arm. You may place a pillow between your ear and your arm so that the head is at the right angle to the spine.
- Bend both legs in front of you at an angle of just under 90°.
- Use your right arm to support yourself in front.
- Throughout the exercise keep lifting the waist off the floor and maintaining the length in the trunk.
- If you are lucky enough to lack any natural padding round your hip, you may find it uncomfortable to lie like this. If so, just put a small piece of foam underneath your hip.

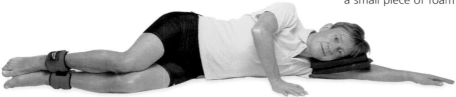

Starting position for Abductor Lifts

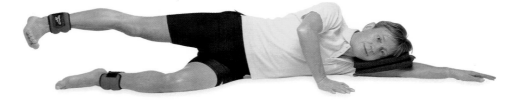

Full position

Action

1 Zip up and hollow (stay zipped and hollowed throughout), straighten you top leg so that it is in a line with your hip – about 12 centimetres off the floor. Be careful not to take it behind you! Rotate the leg in slightly from the hip, the pelvis stays still, and flex the foot towards your face.

2 Breathe out as you slowly lift the leg about another 15 centimetres, then breathe in and lower.

3 Raise and lower the leg ten times, without returning it to the floor.

4 Bend the leg to rest on the bent one underneath.

5 Turn over and repeat on the other side, or complete the other leg weight exercises and then turn over.

Watchpoints

- Keep zipping and hollowing so that you protect the lower back and prevent it from arching or the waist from dropping down to the floor.
- Lengthen the heel as far away as possible from the hip . . . long, long leg.
- Keep the rotation inward from the hip, be careful not to turn it in just from the ankle.
- Keep lifting the waist off the floor and lengthening in the body . . . long, long waist.
- Your pelvis should remain absolutely still, do not allow it to roll forward or rock round.
- Don't forget to keep the upper body open, shoulder blades down into your back.
- Do not allow yourself to roll forward.

Twenty Lifts

A more advanced version of the above, and one which requires a very strong centre.

Aim

To work the gluteals, especially gluteus medius.

Action

1 Follow the directions above, but this time bring the top straight leg in front of you. Aim to have the leg extended at right angles to you (work up to this).

2 Now raise and lower the leg twenty times keeping it at hip height and moving it about 12 centimetres up and down, zipping and hollowing all the time.

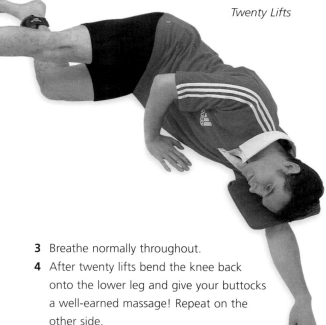

Twenty Lifts

3 Breathe normally throughout.

4 After twenty lifts bend the knee back onto the lower leg and give your buttocks a well-earned massage! Repeat on the other side.

Adductor Lifts

Aim
To tone the inner thigh muscles. To learn pelvic stability.

Equipment
As for Abductor Lifts (page 130) plus a large pillow.

Starting Position
- Lay on your left side as for Abductor Lifts, but now bend your top knee and rest it on top of a large pillow. The idea is for your pelvis to stay square and not drop forward.
- Stretch the bottom leg away a little in front of you, turning it out from the hip joint. Point or flex the foot, either is fine.

Action
1 Breathe in wide and full to prepare.
2 Keeping the leg turned out from the hip, long and straight, breathe out, zip up and hollow (stay zipped and hollowed now) and slowly raise the underneath leg. Keep lengthening it away. Do not allow your waist to sink into the floor, keep working it.
3 Breathe in as you lower the leg.
4 Repeat up to twenty times on each side.

Watchpoints
- Keep zipping and hollowing throughout.
- Don't let the waist sag, keep lengthening it.
- Check that you are moving the whole leg together and not just twisting from the knee.
- Don't let your foot sickle (curl) round to help you come up further. The action must be in the inside of the thigh.
- Check that your upper body stays open, shoulder blades down, do not roll forward.

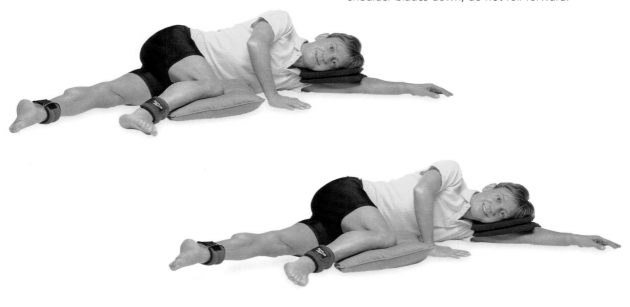

Ankle Circles on the Wall

Aim

To mobilize and strengthen the ankle joints. To work the muscles of the lower leg. To improve circulation. To stretch the hamstrings.

There is no elegant way to get into this position but try wriggling up to the wall on your side and then swing your legs up the wall (stabilizing of course). The closer you are to the wall, the greater the stretch on your hamstrings so if they are still a little tight then leave a gap between the skirting board and your tailbone – you can also have your knees bent. The main thing is that you are in neutral with the tailbone down on the floor.

Take note: Stop if you feel any strange sensations in your legs.

Starting Position

- Lie with your buttocks as close to the wall as is comfortable, with your legs up the wall, in parallel and hip-width apart.
- Now check that you are square to the wall and not at an angle.
- Your pelvis is in neutral.
- You may have your head on a flat pillow if necessary.

Action

1 Keeping the legs completely still, rotate the feet outwards, circling from the ankle joints themselves. You should be circling very, very slowly and as far as you can.
2 Repeat ten circles in each direction.

Watchpoints

- Don't just twiddle the toes round, work from the ankle joints.
- When we say keep the legs still, we mean still! And in parallel!

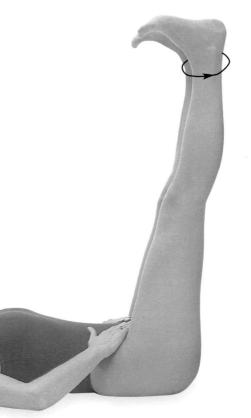

Standing Quadriceps Stretch

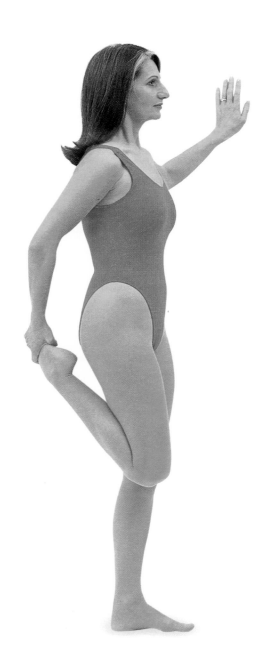

Aim

To stretch the front of the thighs while maintaining correct body alignment.

This is a complementary stretch to the Side-lying Quadricep and Hip Flexor Stretch on page 84. As always alignment is crucial so *do not allow the back to arch!*

Please take advice if you have a knee injury.

Equipment

A scarf (optional, see watchpoints below).

Starting Position

- Stand alongside the wall placing your left hand on the wall for support and remembering all the directions for standing correctly (page 56).

Action

1 Breathe in to prepare and lengthen up through the spine.
2 Breathe out, zip up and hollow and bend the right knee so that you can clasp the ankle. As you do so, check that you have not arched or bowed your back, it must stay neutral. Imagine there is a small weight attached to your tailbone to help keep the length at the base of the spine.

3 Now gently pull the knee towards your buttock, keeping the knee still and in line with your other leg. Do not take it too far back. Keep lengthening from the top of your head to your tailbone.

4 Hold the stretch, breathing normally for thirty seconds. Repeat twice on each leg.

Watchpoints

- If you know that you are not flexible or have a knee problem, use a long scarf and place it over the front of the foot to help. Hold the scarf with the hand and gently bring the foot towards your bottom.

- The most common mistake made with this exercise is to allow the pelvis to shift as the leg bends back. Keep the tailbone lengthening downwards towards the floor and keep the natural curves of the spine without arching the back.

Chalk Circle

Aim

To open the upper body and sides, stretching out the pectoral muscles of the chest. To rotate the spine safely with stability, working from a strong centre.

This exercise has the most wonderful feel-good factor. Perfect at the end of a bad day, or even a good day!!

Please consult your practitioner before starting this exercise if you have a shoulder or disc injury.

Starting Position

- Lie on your side with a pillow under your head – a bed pillow is perfect.
- Have your back in a straight line but curl your knees up to hip level.
- Extend your arms in front of you, in line with your shoulders, palms together.

Action

1 Breathe in to prepare and lengthen through the spine.
2 Breathe out, zip up and hollow.
3 Imagining you have a piece of chalk in your hand, reach the top arm beyond the lower arm, taking your hand above you over your head. Allow your head to move naturally, following the opening movement of the

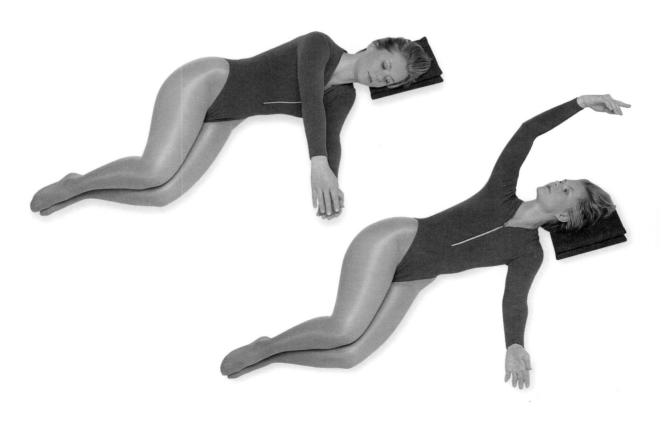

shoulders. The knees stay together and the centre strong.

4 Breathe normally now, reach your hand right round as if you are drawing a circle on the floor. It will pass behind you, down over your buttocks and back up to join the other hand.

5 Repeat five times on each side. The aim is to keep the hand in contact with the floor but, as that's difficult, please work within your comfort range.

Watchpoints

- As you allow your head to follow the movement, take care that you do not shorten the back of the neck, it should stay released.
- Keep zipping and hollowing.
- Do not allow the back to arch.
- Keep the knees on the ground, even if it means that your hand does not touch the floor.
- Do not force the arm at all.

This is the last exercise in the Intermediate Programme. You may like to finish with the Relaxation on page 90. Well done!

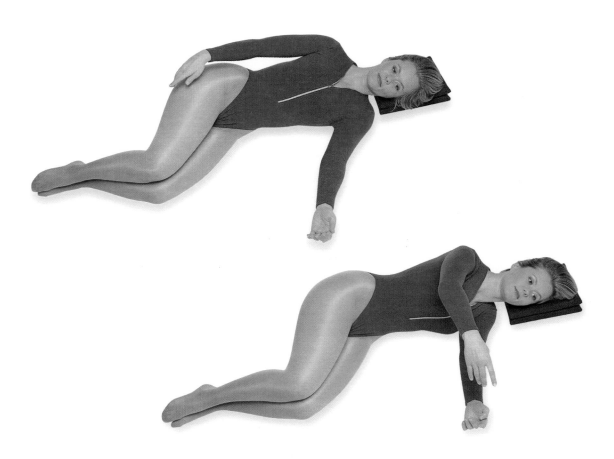

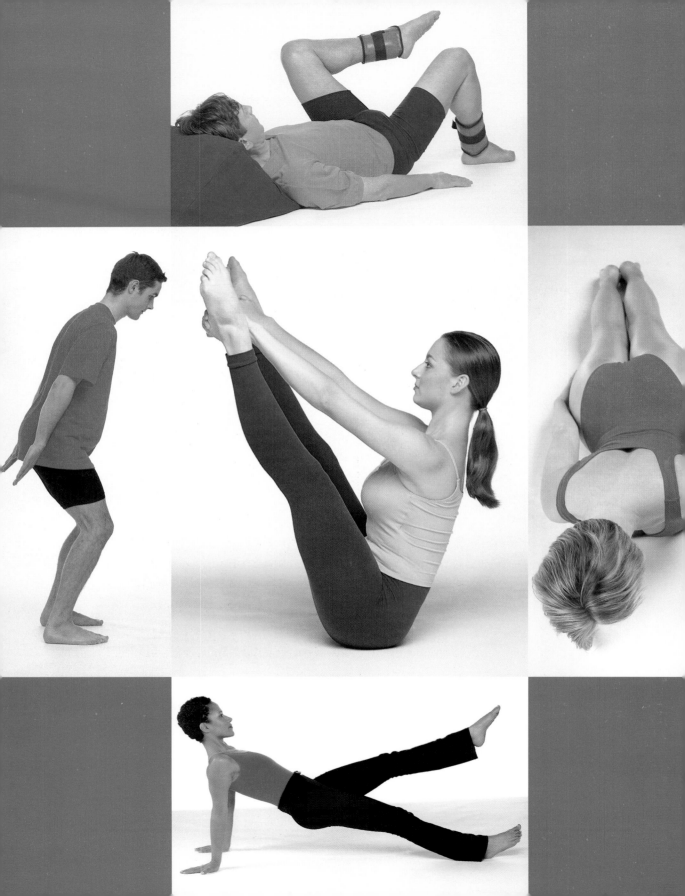

The
Advanced
Programme

Now we really moving, and moving naturally and easily, the Pilates Way.

This final section will bring together all the skills you have mastered, all the Eight Principles. The classical exercises will both challenge and stimulate your mind and your body. Some are very difficult so,

if you find you are struggling, please be sensible and return to the Intermediate Programme until you are stronger. If you push yourself too far, the wrong muscles will work. You may always add some exercises from the Beginner's and Intermediate Programmes.

Advanced Warm Up: Walking on the Spot

Aim

To warm up the body, especially the muscles. To stimulate the circulation.

Warm Up

Action

1 Stand with your feet just closer than hip-width apart and start to walk on the spot.
2 Come up onto the ball of one foot and transfer your weight onto the other foot. Keep your pelvis level and your waist long. Make sure that your knee bends over the centre of your foot and does not deviate inwards or outwards. Now change sides, transferring the weight. Keep lengthening upwards.
3 Keep walking like this for two minutes.

Watchpoints

• When walking on the spot, keep checking your ankle, knee and foot alignment. If they are wrong, it may be better for you to practise the foot exercises on pages 75–6 for a little longer.

Roll Downs with Balance

Aim

Releasing tension in the spine, the shoulders and the upper body. To mobilize the spine, creating

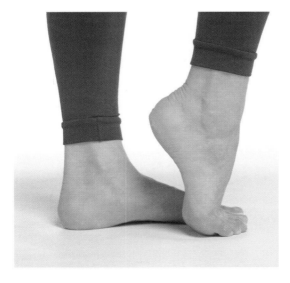

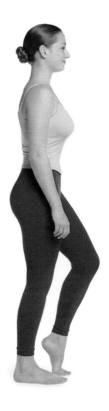

flexibility and strength and achieving segmental control. To teach correct use of stabilizing abdominals. To improve balance skills and proprioception (body awareness).

Please take advice if you have a back problem (see below), especially if disc related.

Starting Position

- Stand with your feet hip-width apart and in parallel, your weight evenly balanced on both feet. Check that you are not rolling your feet in or out. Soften your knees.
- Find your neutral pelvis position but keep the tailbone lengthening down.

Action

1 Breathe in to prepare and lengthen up through the spine, release the head and neck.
2 Breathe out, zip up and hollow, drop your chin onto your chest and allow the weight of your

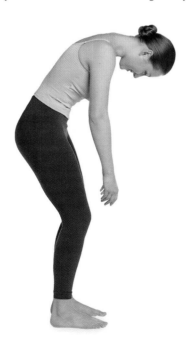

head to make you slowly roll forward, head released, arms hanging, centre strong, knees soft.
3 Breathe in as you hang, really letting your head and arms hang.
4 Breathe out, still firmly zipped up and hollowed, as you drop your tailbone down, directing your pubic bone forward. Rotate your pelvis backwards as you slowly come up to standing tall, rolling through the spine bone by bone.
5 When you have unfurled, lengthen up through the spine and come up onto the balls of your feet.
6 Slowly lower the heels down maintaining the length in the body.
7 Repeat six times.

Watchpoints

- Make sure you go down centrally and do not sway over to one side. When you are down, check where your hands are in relation to your feet.
- Do not roll the feet in or out. Keep the weight evenly balanced and try not to lean forward onto the front of your feet or back onto the heels.
- Balance – keep using your centre, keep lengthening and do keep correct postural alignment, that is try not to pitch the body forwards or backwards.

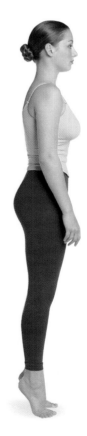

The Scapular Squeeze

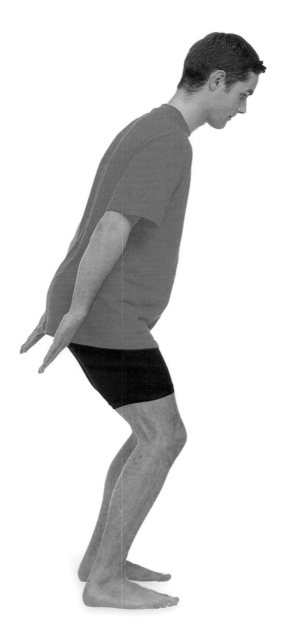

Aim

To strengthen the stabilizing muscles between and underneath the shoulder blades, opening the chest. To strengthen the back of the upper arms. To lengthen the spine.

A wonderful exercise for the upper back and the upper arms where, unfortunately, we all tend to get a bit flabby! Not any more, if you do this exercise and the arm-weights series!!

Starting Position

- Stand, feet in parallel, hip-width apart. Your knees are bent directly over your feet.
- Now pivot forward on your hips as if you are skiing downhill, your head, neck and back remain in one piece. Look at a spot on the floor in front of you at a distance that keeps the back of your neck free from tension and the top of the head lengthening away (see photo). If you look too close, your head will drop; too far away and you shorten the back of the neck.
- Take your arms, behind you and to the sides, the palms face upwards.

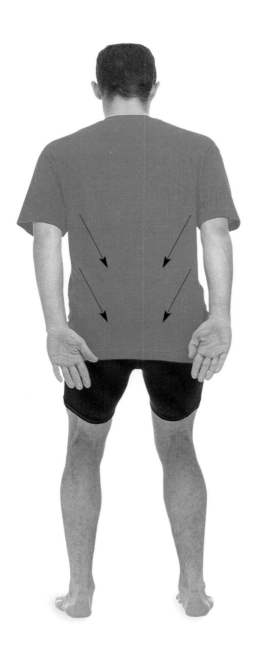

Action

1 Breathe in to prepare and lengthen up through the spine.

2 Breathe out, zip up and hollow and slide the shoulder blades down before you squeeze them together. Your arms are also squeezing towards each other as if the thumbs want to meet.

3 Breathe in and hold.

4 Breathe out and release the arms.

5 Repeat five times before returning to upright. When coming back to an upright position, keep lengthening your back and head away and return to a balanced way of standing without locking your knees.

Watchpoints

• Keep your gaze on your spot on the floor.

• Check your neck, keep it released and long.

• Think of the tailbone lengthening downwards away from the top of your head.

• Keep the knees softly bent and over your feet.

• Make sure that you are feeling this exercise between the shoulder blades and also at the back of your upper arms. Do not lock the arms, they are straight but not locked.

Spine Curls into Curl Ups

Aim

To learn how to wheel the spine, vertebra by vertebra, achieving synchronous segmental control, using the stabilizing muscles. To work the abdominals.

Combining two exercises in this fashion helps to reinforce good movement patterns and to make you really aware of moving correctly.

Equipment

A plump pillow.

Starting Position

- Lie on your back with your feet flat on the floor, in parallel, just a few centimetres apart and about 30 centimetres from your buttocks.
- Place the pillow between your knees.
- Your arms are relaxed down by your side, palms down.

Action

1 Breathe in to prepare.
2 Breathe out, zip up and hollow and curl the tailbone off the floor just a little.
3 Breathe in then breathe out, zip up and hollow and slowly curl back down lengthening out the spine.
4 Breathe in then out, zip up and hollow and peel a little more of the spine off the floor.
5 Breathe in then out as you place the spine back down, bone by bone.
6 Repeat five times.
7 On the sixth repeat, when you are fully curled up, breathe in and take both arms soft and wide above your head.
8 As you breathe out, still zipped and hollowed, slowly return the spine to the floor bone by bone.

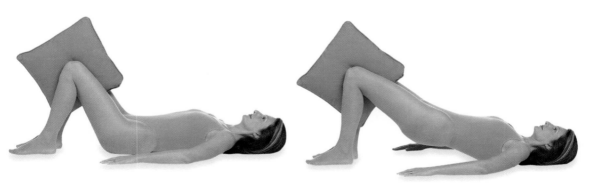

1. Starting position　　　*2. Action 4*

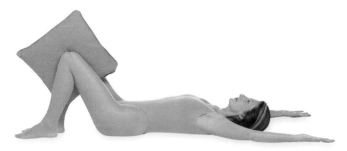

3. Action 8

9 Breathe in and bring both arms up to chest level.

10 As you breathe out, gently curl the upper body off the floor lengthening through the fingertips, engaging the shoulder blades down into your back. Do not tuck your pelvis.

11 Breathe in and lower.

12 Repeat five times.

Watchpoints

- Keep the weight even on both feet and try not to let the feet roll in or out.
- Keep your neck long and soft.
- It is very tempting to tuck the pelvis as you curl the upper body off the floor in the final movement – don't! Remember everything you learnt for Curl Ups on page 78.

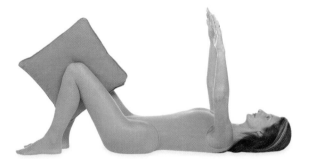

4. Action 9

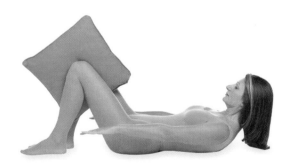

5. Action 10

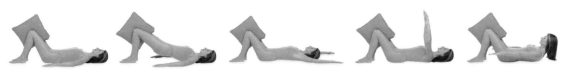

1. Starting positon *2.* *3.* *4.* *5.*

Advanced Hip Rolls

Aim

To stretch and work the waist, to strengthen the oblique abdominals (see diagram page 79). To achieve a safe rotation of the spine, with segmental control. To promote awareness of the shoulder blades, using the stabilizing muscles. To learn co-ordination skills. To challenge stability by lengthening the lever.

By extending the leg, it becomes a longer lever which requires you to really use your abdominals to stay in control. We are looking here for rotation with stability. The ability to rotate the spine is the first movement we tend to lose as we grow old. There is a lot to think about with this exercise, which is great as we are trying to train the mind as well as the body! Focus on:

- Using the lower abdominals throughout.
- Peeling each part of your back off the floor in turn – first your buttocks leave the floor, then the hips, then the waist and finally the back of the ribs. Then as you return to the centre, place each part of your back on the floor in reverse order – the ribs, the waist, the hips, the buttocks.
- As you turn the palm down, think of the shoulder blade setting itself down into your back.

Please take advice if you have a disc-related injury. If you have had a whiplash injury, keep your head in the centre.

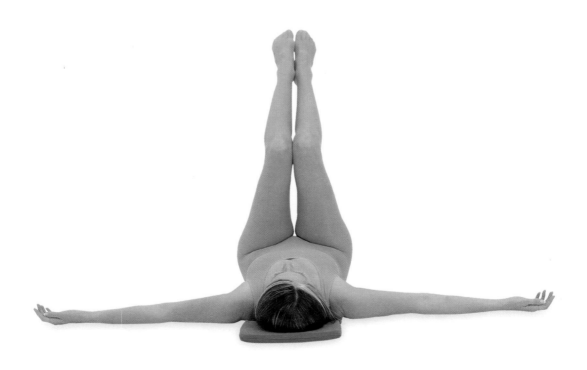

Starting Position

- Lie on your back, arms out to the side, palms up.
- Your knees should be up towards your chest but in line with your hips. Your thighs will be at right angles to your body. Your feet are softly pointed.

Action

1 Breathe in wide and full to prepare.

2 As you breathe out, zip up and hollow and slowly lower your legs towards the floor on your left side, turning your head to the right and your right palm down. Keep the right shoulder down on the ground.

3 Keep the knees in line.

4 Stay zipped and hollowed throughout.

5 Breathe in and breathe out, and slowly straighten the right leg. Use this strong centre to bring your legs back to the middle – the right leg stays extended. The head returns to the middle, the palm turns up again.

6 Breathe in and then out, and repeat the twisting movement to the opposite side.

7 Repeat ten times to each side.

Watchpoints

- Keep the opposite shoulder firmly down on the floor.
- Keep the knees in line. Don't go too far unless you can control it.
- Use the abdominals at all times – feel as though you are moving the legs from the stomach.
- It is a sideways lateral movement, don't deviate.
- Do not force the neck the opposite way, allow it to roll comfortably and keep long.

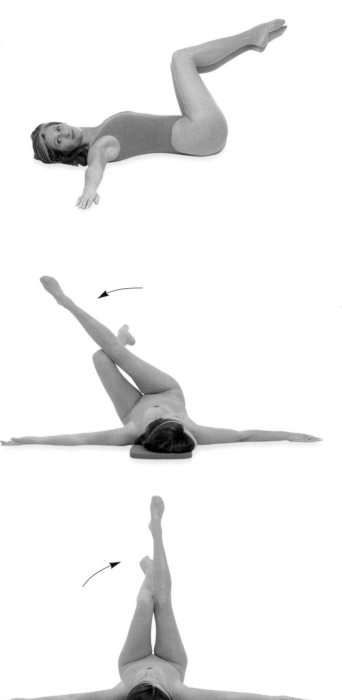

The Full Hundred

Aim

To learn how to stabilize the trunk and co-ordinate breathing, centring and limb movement. To strengthen the abdominals. To work the deep neck flexors. To stimulate the circulation. To improve stamina. To work the inner thighs and deep buttock muscles, especially the stabilizers – the gluteus medius and the external hip rotators.

This is a classical exercise which you should find really invigorating! You should have mastered stages 1–4 (page 120).

Starting Position

- Lie with your knees bent up onto your chest, arms down by your side palms down.
- Allow your head to roll gently from side to side.

Action

1 Breathe in wide and full to prepare.
2 Breathe out, zip up and hollow (you will stay zipped and hollowed throughout), tuck the chin in slightly and curl the upper body off the floor at the same time straightening the legs into the air in parallel. Reach through the fingertips engaging the shoulder blades down into the back.

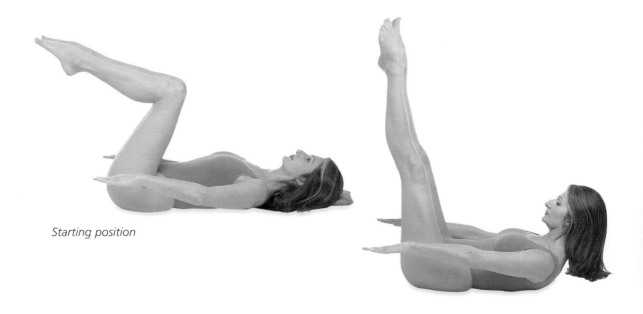

Starting position

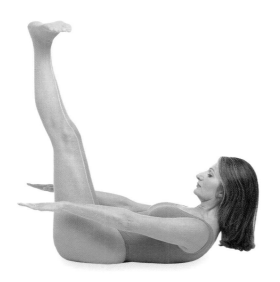

Watchpoints

- The abdominals continue to work throughout, you should feel the inner thighs squeezing against each other and the pelvic floor engaging.
- Keep lengthening the fingers away from your ears, the shoulder blades stay down into your back.
- Keep the upper body wide and open, do not close your shoulders in.
- Please come down if you feel your neck is straining.

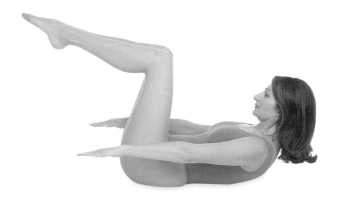

3 Turn your legs out now from the hips and flex the feet, lengthening through the heels so that you feel the stretch on the inside of the legs. Keep your legs anchored into the hips. Squeeze your inner thighs together and engage the pelvic floor. Breathe in for five beats of the arm, out for five beats, pumping the arms as they reach towards your feet.

4 After one hundred beats, bend your knees and curl back down.

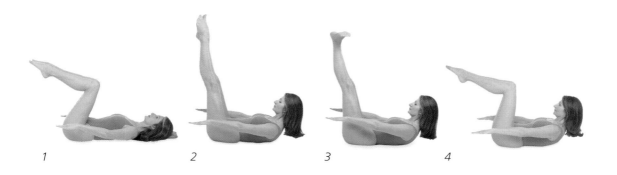

1   2   3   4

The Seal (Stages One and Two)

Aim

To learn co-ordination and control. To work the abdominals. To massage the spine. To entertain on-lookers! An exercise best done in a darkened room with the curtains pulled!

Please take advice if you have a spinal or disc-related problem and avoid if you have osteoporosis or a scoliosis.

Stage One: Rolling Like a Ball

Aim

To prepare for The Seal.

Starting Position

- Sit with your feet on the mat and hold both legs firmly under the thighs.

Action

1 Breathe in to prepare.
2 Breathe out, zip up and hollow and roll backwards, keeping your knees bent, your chin tucked in and your body curled up like a ball.
3 Breathe in and roll back up to sitting.
4 Repeat 5 times.

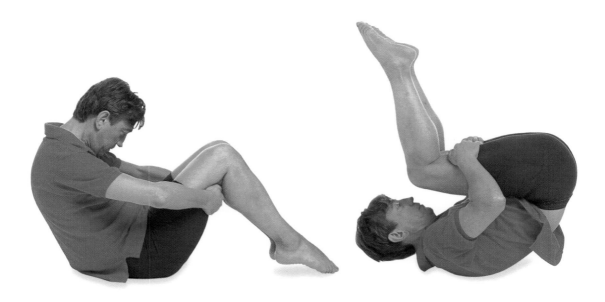

Stage Two: The Seal

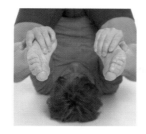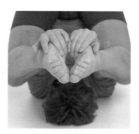

Starting Position

- Sit with your feet on your mat. Have your heels together and the toes apart. Take your arms in front of you and down through the inside of your legs and round the back of your ankles to hold the ankles in the front. See the photo!
- Gently tuck in your chin.

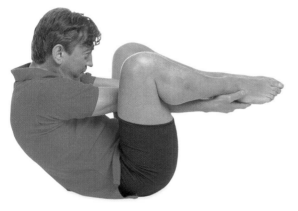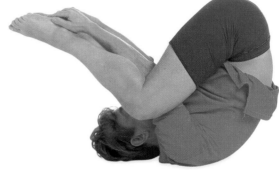

Action

1 Breathe in to prepare.
2 Breathe out, zip up and hollow and roll backwards. When back, flap your feet together twice like flippers.
3 Breathe in, still zipped and hollowed, as you roll upright again. Don't put your feet on the floor, but flap them again like flippers.
4 Repeat five times.

Now you know why it's called The Seal!!!

Watchpoints

- Use your abdominals throughout.
- Do not roll too far back.
- Keep your chin tucked in.

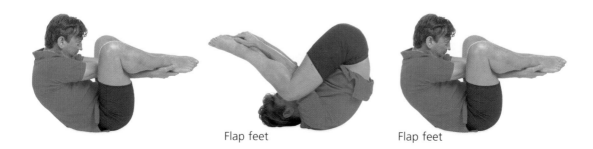

Flap feet   Flap feet

Spine Rolls

Aim

To mobilize the full length of the spine. To achieve segmental control as the stabilizing muscles engage.

This exercise requires good hamstring length!

Do not even think about attempting this exercise if you suffer from back or neck problems!

Starting Position

- Lie in the Relaxation Position.
- Bring one leg at the time into the chest, engaging the lower abdominals when lifting. Straighten the legs at a right angle to the floor, feet softly pointed and legs turned out.

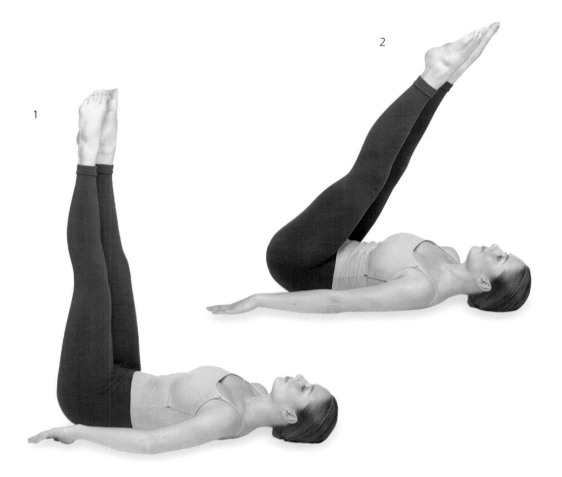

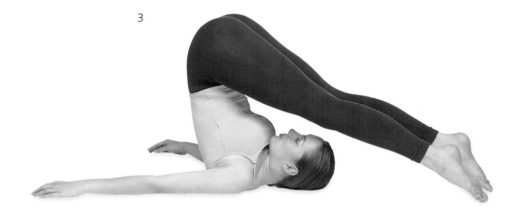

3

Action

1 Breathe out, zip up and hollow and lower the straight legs into your chest.

2 Still engaging the lower abdominals, start to roll back, bringing your knees towards your nose until eventually you touch the floor with your feet behind your head – don't worry if you can't! This movement should be smooth and controlled.

3 Breathe in to turn the legs in parallel and open them shoulder-width apart.

4 Breathe out, still zipping and hollowing and slowly roll one vertebrae at a time back onto the mat until you return to the starting position.

5 Repeat five times.

Watchpoints

• Keep your arms, shoulders and neck relaxed, especially when rolling back down!

• Do not roll onto the neck! Keep the neck long.

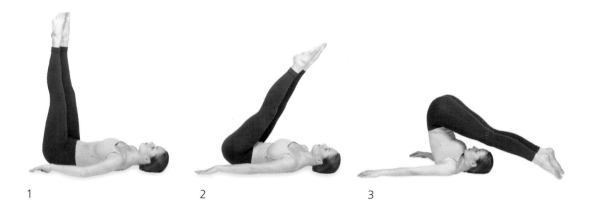

1   2   3

Advanced Double Leg Stretch

Aim

To improve co-ordination skills. To strengthen the stabilizing muscles of the abdomen and the deep neck flexors. To increase stamina. To open the upper body and work the shoulders. To work the inner thighs and the deep muscles of the buttocks, especially gluteus medius and the external hip rotators.

This is the Pilates Method at its finest. A complex, choreographed sequence which conditions the entire body, using mind-body skills. The right muscles are activated to achieve the movements: the stabilizers working as they should; the mobilizers working as they should; free, graceful movements with stability. The instructions may seem lengthy, but this is because this exercise requires you to control every aspect of your body.

A word about the breathing. You will notice an unusual breathing pattern for this exercise. You inhale as you curl off the floor. Why? We tend to use the out breath at the hardest part of an exercise, when we need most stability from the deep abdominals. The hardest part of this exercise is when the arms are taken back in a wide sweep.

The Leg Action

Let's just take a separate look at the leg action – you are straightening the legs into the air in a turned out position. In the starting position, the toes are touching, the heels are apart. As you straighten the legs, you move from toes to heels and then, when straight, you flex the feet.

Starting Position

- Lie with your knees bent, they are open from the hip. Your toes are just touching but your heels are apart.
- Have your hands resting on the outside of your knees. Your elbows are open, breastbone soft, shoulder blades down into your back.
- Gently roll your head from side to side to release the neck.

Advanced double leg stretch sequence

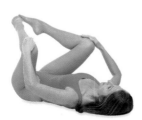 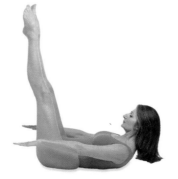 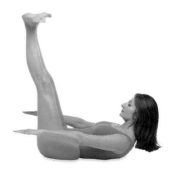

1. Starting position   *2*   *3*

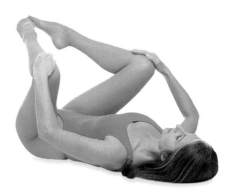

Starting and finishing position

Action

1 Breath in to prepare and then out, zip up and hollow. These core muscles should stay engaged now throughout the exercise.

2 Breathe in and slowly curl your upper body from the floor, gently tucking in the chin. At the same time straighten your legs so that they are turned out from the hips.

3 Flex the feet and lengthen up the inside of your legs to the heels. Squeeze the inner thighs together. Your fingers are lengthening away from you just below the knees on the outside of your thighs.

4 Breathe out, still zipped and hollowed and take your arms up in a wide sweep to the level of your ears, not behind. Keep the natural curve of the arms.

5 Breathe in as the arms circle back round to alongside the thighs again.

6 Breathe out as you slowly lower your head back down onto the floor, bending the knees so that they are back in the starting position.

7 Repeat ten times.

Watchpoints

- Do not allow the abdominals to bulge at all during the exercise.
- Keep your neck long, the superficial muscles released.
- With the legs turned out and straight, make sure that you anchor the head of your thigh bones into the hips.
- Do not allow the legs to fall away.
- Do not take your arms behind the level of your ears.

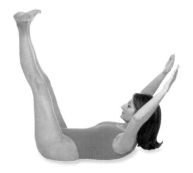

4

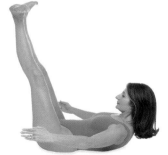

5

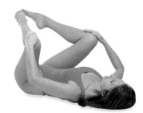

6

Dart into Side Bend

Aim

To strengthen the back, especially the muscles in the mid back and the waist.

This is a lovely variation to The Dart on page 70.

Starting Position

- Lie on your front, legs together, feet softly pointed.
- Your forehead is resting on the floor or an a flat pillow, arms alongside, elbows soft.

Action

1 Breathe in to prepare. Breathe out, zip up and hollow, engaging the muscles of the inner thighs, to bring the legs together. Maintain this throughout the exercise.

2 Breathe in and out, still zippped up, move your palms so that they are facing towards the thighs bringing the arms off the floor, then reach towards the feet. Imagine your shoulder blades gliding down the back. As a result the head will lift off the floor in line with your body, long neck, face down.

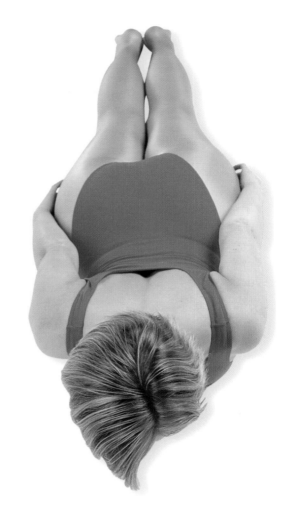

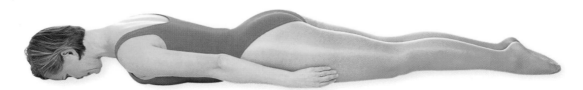

Starting position

3 Breathe in in this position, still zipping and hollowing.

4 Breathe out and bend from the waist, one arm glides down the leg. Make sure that you do not change the angle of your head on the spine. The neck stays long.

5 Breathe in to return to centre.

6 Breathe out, keep zipping and hollowing and repeat on the other side.

7 Breathe in to return to the middle and gently release back down, this time turning your head the other way.

8 Repeat six times to each side.

9 When you have finished this exercise, come onto all fours and back into the Rest Position (page 73), do not do this if you have a knee problem.

Watchpoints

- Don't forget to support your lower back by zipping and hollowing.
- Do not come up too high.
- When side bending, do not rotate or twist the back but keep the movement on one plane.
- Do not clench your buttock muscles. Use the muscles of the inner thigh to create a stable base.

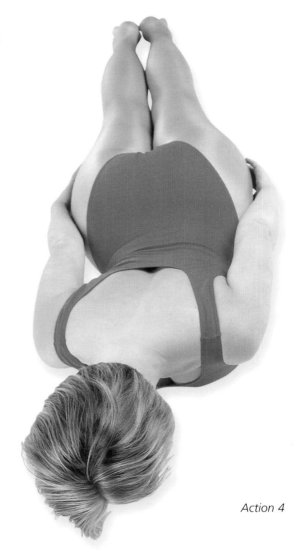

Action 4

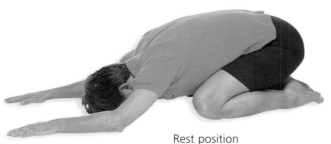

Rest position

Advanced Table Top

Aim

To mobilize the spine, strengthen the abdominals and the buttock muscles. To learn balance and control.

Starting Position

- Kneel on all fours, your hands directly beneath your shoulders, your knees beneath your hips.
- Check that your pelvis is neutral, the natural curve maintained.

Action

1 Breathe in to prepare as you lengthen the spine from the top of your head to your tailbone.
2 Breathe out, zip up and hollow and bring your left knee forward towards your head, curling your head to meet the knee while arching the back up.

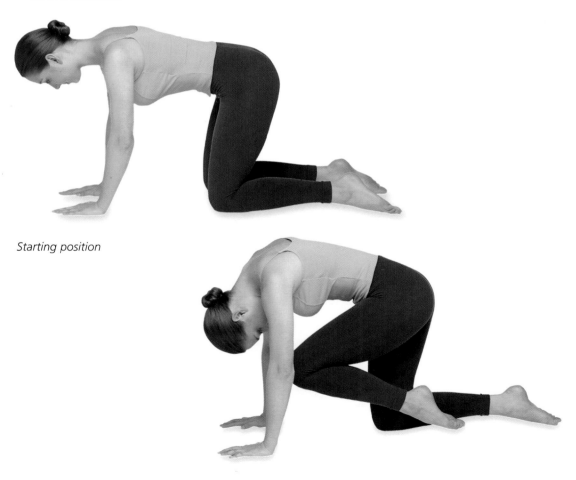

Starting position

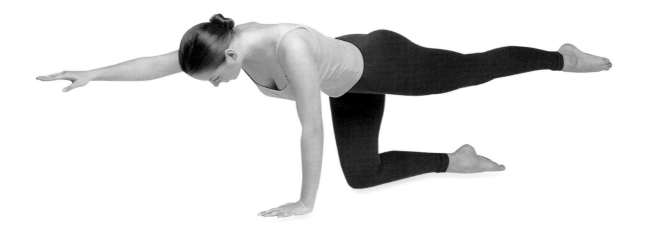

3 Breathe out, still zipping and hollowing and straighten the leg, extending it along the floor until the knee is straight, then lift it behind you no higher than your buttocks. At the same time lift your right arm and extend it in front of you. Do not twist the pelvis – keep it square to you.

4 Breathe in and hold.

5 Breathe out, still zipping and hollowing and bend the knee in again curling the head to meet it.

6 Repeat five times on each side.

7 When you have finished, bring your feet together and sit back on your heels in the Rest Position – do not do this if you have a knee injury (see page 73).

Watchpoints

Remember everything you learnt in the single versions of Table Top (page 110).

• Stay zipped and hollowed throughout

• Keep the leg movements slow and controlled.

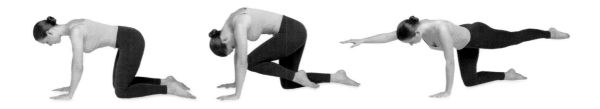

Scissors and Scissors with Co-ordination

Aim

To strengthen the abdominals and improve the flexibility of hamstrings and co-ordination.

Starting Position

- Lie on the mat.
- Bring your knees bent onto your chest and take hold of the right leg behind the thigh.

Action

1 Breathe in wide and full to prepare.
2 Breathe out, zip up and hollow (stay zipped and hollowed throughout now), curl the head and shoulders off the mat. Keep the breastbone soft.
3 Breathe in and straighten both legs up into the air, toes softly pointed. You are still holding the right leg behind the thigh.
4 Breathe out, lengthen the left leg towards the floor, stopping just above it.
5 Breathe in and raise the leg as straight as possible.
6 Breathe out, change arms and legs and lower the right leg.
7 Repeat ten times on each leg. Aim to cross over like scissors. Stay zipped and hollowed throughout.

Watchpoints

- Long, long legs. Keep lengthening away.
- Strong centre at all times.
- Upper body stays open, shoulder blades down, neck released.

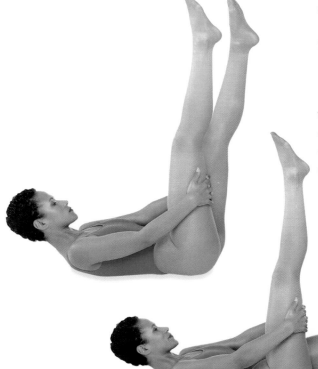

Scissors with Co-ordination

This version requires cast-iron stomach muscles – you have been warned!!!

Action

1 Follow the steps above but repeat the movement only twice.
2 Breathe out and lower both legs in parallel to about 45°. Extend the arms through the fingertips along the torso.
3 Breathe in to prepare.
4 Breathe out and open and close the legs rapidly slightly wider than shoulder-width. Focus on your inner thighs.

5 Breathe in and raise the legs back to the starting position, as in Step 3 above.
6 Repeat the full set of movements up to four times.

Watchpoints

- Keep zipping and hollowing throughout, pelvis neutral, the tailbone lengthening away. The full version requires very strong abdominals!
- The upper body stays soft and open, your shoulder blades are down into your back.
- Keep your legs as straight as possible.

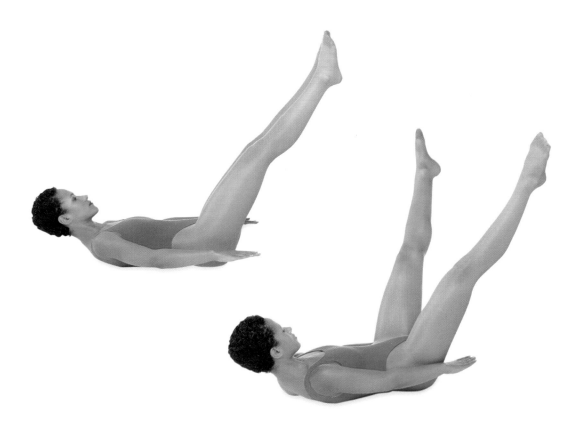

Side Kicks into Arabesque

Aim

To stretch and strengthen the hip flexors. To increase core stability and awareness of trunk alignment.

You can perform this exercise with parallel or turned out legs.

This is a difficult exercise to do correctly. Should you experience any back pain during this movement, discontinue immediately.

1. Starting position

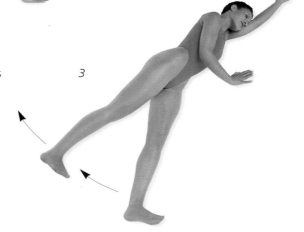

2

3

Starting Position

- Lie on the mat on one side, your head resting on an outstretched arm. The other hand helps to stabilize one shoulder on top of the other by being placed in front of your chest at a right angle.
- Hip stays over hip, waist long and slightly off the mat.
- Bring the straight legs slightly in front of the torso, feet flexed.

Action

1 Breathe in wide and full to prepare.
2 Breathe out, zip up and hollow and lift the top leg to hip level.
3 Breathe in, stay zipped and hollowed and kick the leg forward as far as you can without losing neutral pelvis. The waist stays long and slightly off the mat.
4 Breathe out. While maintaining a strong centre kick the leg behind you. Do not let the back arch or the ribcage flare.
5 Repeat five times to each side.

Watchpoints

- The moving leg should not drop below hip level when it kicks forward or backward.
- Keep a sense of lengthening through the crown of your head and tailbone.
- Keep your alignment, lifting from the waist. Do not allow the waist to sink.
- Do not hollow the lower back or stick your ribs out when the leg goes back.

Oblique Single Leg Stretch (Criss Cross)

Aim

To work the abdominals – especially the obliques – while challenging co-ordination and core stability.

A powerful exercise that hits the spot. You'll need strong abdominals to do this one correctly. There is another variation called Criss Cross in the Series of Five on page 174.

Starting Position

- Lie on your back, draw your knees up onto your chest, the toes just touching – but not the heels. Keep your feet softly pointed.
- Clasp your hands behind your head. The elbows stay open.

Action

1 Breathe in wide and full to prepare.
2 Breathe out, zip up and hollow as you curl up, softening the breastbone and taking the right shoulder in the direction of your left knee. The upper body stays open, the elbows in line. At the same time straighten the right leg, extending it in parallel at an angle of about 45° to the floor.
3 Breathe out, still zipped and hollowed and curl the left shoulder towards the right bent knee, extending the left leg away.
4 Repeat ten times to each side.

Watchpoints

- Make sure that the shoulder, and not the elbow, comes across towards the bent knee.
- Keep the elbows in line, do not allow them to come forward – it is your shoulder that is directed towards the knee. In this way, the upper body stays open.
- Stay neutral please.

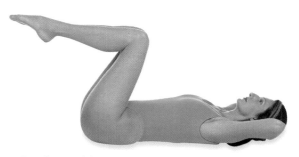

Starting position

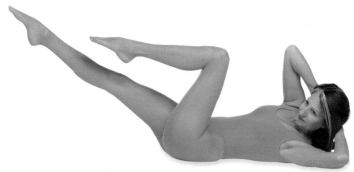

Full position

Open Leg Rocker (Stages One and Two)

Aim

This exercise tests and improves both your ability to centre and your sense of balance.

Please note that you should be able to do the Spine Rolls on page 152 and The Seal on page 150 before you attempt this exercise. Make sure that you are fully warmed up and that your hamstrings are stretched before you begin to attempt Open Leg Rocker.

Clear all valuable furniture and belongings out of the way and turn the mobile off!

We have given you a preparation exercise and then the full exercise.

Stage One

Starting Position

- Sit tall on your sitting bones, bend one knee at a time, feet softly pointed. Hold onto the inside of your ankles. Balance in this position by zipping and hollowing.

Action

1 Breathe in wide and full to prepare and lengthen through the spine.
2 Breathe out, zip up and hollow and straighten the legs into a V-shape, keeping the back as straight as possible. Try to keep your arms as straight as possible without locking the elbows. Should you not be able to straighten your legs by holding onto the ankles, try holding onto the calves instead.
3 Breathe in to fold the legs.
4 Repeat six times.

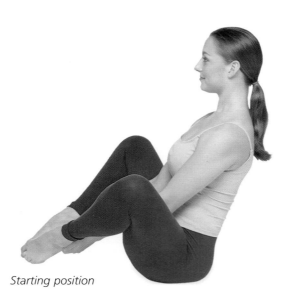

Starting position

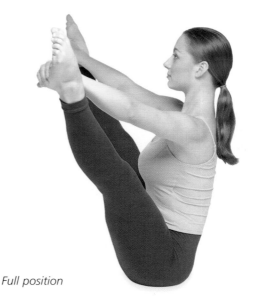

Full position

Stage Two

Action

1 Follow steps 1 and 2 above.
2 Breathe out, zip up and hollow and tilt your pelvis backwards (into the north position) – this is done with control from the abdominals. Your lower back will now be in a C-curve. Still on the same out breath, start rolling back smoothly along the spine.
3 Breathe in to return to the upright position, sitting tall, long back and head straight.
4 Repeat for a maximum of six times before folding the legs.

Watchpoints

- Do not roll onto your neck!
- Balancing with both legs straight requires very good balancing and centring skills, so you must keep zipping and hollowing.
- Try to keep your back as long as possible, ribcage flat.

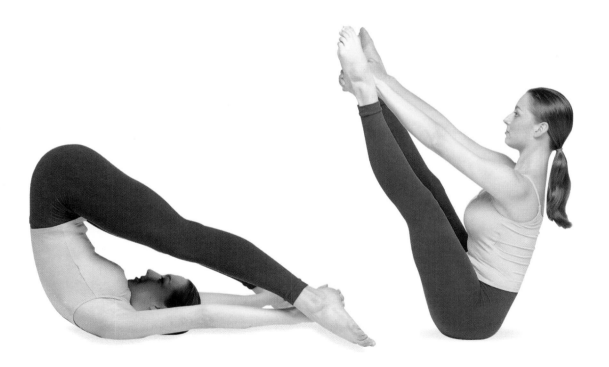

Leg Pulls – Front and Back

Front Leg Pull

Aim
Opens the hip joint and increases strength in the shoulders and lower back.

Starting Position
- As in conventional push ups. Make sure that your body is long and the shoulders down into your back. The fingers point forwards, elbows stay straight but not locked, head in line with the body. Legs are hip-width apart.

Action
1 Breathe in to prepare, stay zipped throughout.
2 Breathe out, zip up and hollow. Press the heels into the floor as far as you can.
3 Breathe in as you lift a leg (keeping foot flexed) towards the ceiling without moving the hips or the back arching. Keep lengthening the head away and the ribcage flat.
4 Breathe out as you lower the leg back to the floor still lengthening through the heel.
5 Repeat on the other leg. Repeat five times with each leg.

Watchpoints
- Maintain both scapular and pelvic stability.
- Keep the back of the neck long and released.
- Don't dip in the middle.

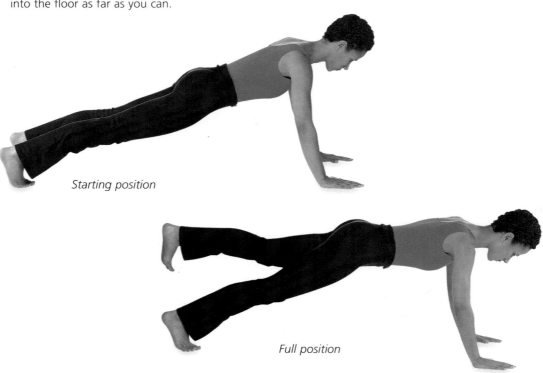

Starting position

Full position

Back Leg Pull

Aim

Stretches the hamstrings, challenges stability, increases hip mobility and strengthens the shoulder girdle.

Starting Position

- Lie on your back.
- Extend the arms below the shoulders, the elbows are straight but not locked. The head, ribcage, hips and heels are in a line, toes pointed and shoulder blades down into the back (see below).

Action

1 Breathe in to prepare.
2 Breathe out, zip up and hollow and stay zipped and hollowed throughout the exercise.
3 Breathe in and kick one leg (foot flexed) to the ceiling. It is important not to lose the alignment, the hips stay up, the pelvis level and the neck and head stay long. Shoulders stay relaxed.
4 Breathe out and point the foot as you slowly lower the leg to the floor.
5 Touch the floor lightly before kicking the same leg again.
6 Repeat five times with each leg.

Watchpoints

- Keep the trunk in a line when the leg kicks up.
- The neck and head especially must stay long.
- Maintain scapular and pelvic stability.
- Do not allow your middle to drop.

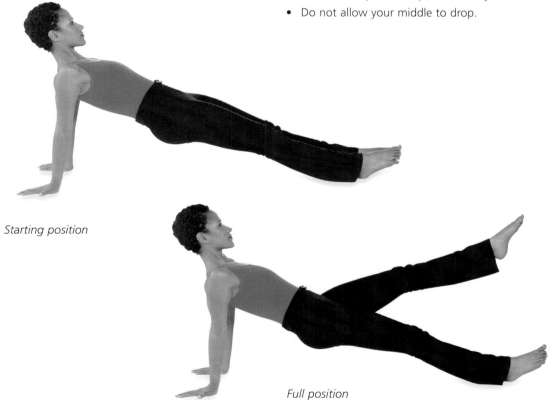

Starting position

Full position

The Saw

Aim

This exercise works on many levels but its main aims are to stretch your spine, sides, inner thighs and hamstrings, while stabilizing.

You will notice that there are a lot of instructions for Step 4. It would be wise to read them through first a couple of times and study the photos before you begin. You should be able to do the Spine Stretch on page 124 comfortably before attempting this exercise

Please note that as this exercise involves bending forward and rotating the spine, anyone with back problems should consult their specialist before attempting it.

Starting Position

- Sit on your sitting bones with your legs in front of you. If you like, you may sit on a rolled up towel. It will help you to keep your pelvis at the right angle.

- Take your legs a comfortable distance apart. Do not force the knees down into the floor, they may remain a little bent if necessary. Have your toes softly pointed until you are very flexible when you can have your feet flexed.

Action

1 Breathe in to prepare and lengthen the spine up an imaginary pole. Bring your arms up to your sides, parallel to the floor like aeroplane wings. Your palms are down. You are reaching through the fingertips. Your shoulder blades stay down into your back.

2 Breathe out, zip up and hollow and rotate your body to the right so that you are facing your right leg.

3 Breathe in and lengthen up again.

4 Breathe out, still zipped and hollowed and rotate to the right some more, at the same time

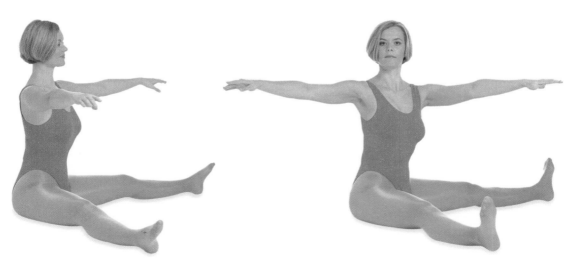

Starting position. Action 1

Action 2/3

reach forward and down so that the edge of your left hand slides down to the outside of the little toe of your right foot. It is as if you are going to saw the toe off! As your left arm reaches forward, stretch your right arm out behind you, raising it as high as possible like a wing, the palm facing backwards. The shoulder blade stays down. Your eyes will now, hopefully, be looking behind you. The back of your neck stays long. Your buttocks are glued to the floor!

5 Take two breaths in this position, then return on the out-breath by reversing the instructions. Remember to lengthen and pause before you return to centre.

6 Repeat five times to each side.

Watchpoints

- Remember to keep zipping and hollowing throughout.
- Both buttocks stay on the floor.
- Your neck stays released.

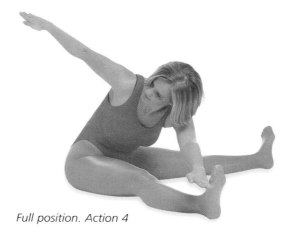

Full position. Action 4

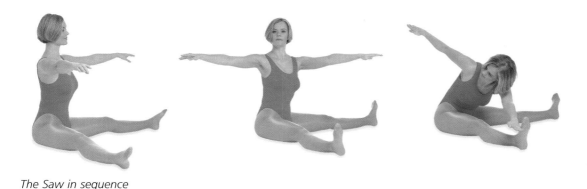

The Saw in sequence

The Leg Weight Series: Passé Développés

Aim

To achieve the correct balance in the leg, hip and buttock muscles. To learn stability of the pelvis. To work the muscles which turn the leg out from the hip (lateral rotators). To achieve control of the muscles round the hip joint.

Normally for this exercise we would use a triangular cushion made from foam which offers just the right amount of support for the spine. If you cannot get hold of one, use a couple of pillows. Otherwise you may lie in the Relaxation Position, with your head supported. Once you have mastered the movements and are stable, you may wear leg weights so that you are toning the muscles.

Remember the exercise Turning Out the Leg in Pelvic Stability on page 40. You are going to do the same action now, turning out the leg from the hip without losing the stability of the pelvis.

Please take advice if you suffer from sciatica.

Equipment

A triangular cushion or large pillow (optional).

Leg weights of 0.5 to 1.5 kilograms each weight. If you have no weights, it is simple to make your own – see page 254.

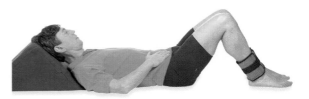

Starting position

Starting Position

- Lie on the cushion or pillows. The idea is that your upper back is supported, but your lower ribcage, waist and pelvis are on the mat. Above all, you should feel comfortable and not scrunched up. You knees are bent hip-width apart and in parallel.
- Otherwise lie in the Relaxation Position.

Action

1 Breathe in to prepare
2 Breathe out, zip up and hollow and fold your knee up, turn it out from the hip, without moving the pelvis.
3 Breathe in, still zipped and hollowed and slowly straighten the leg, keeping it turned out from, and in a line with, your hip. Keep your tailbone on the floor.

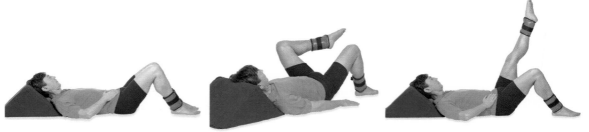

1. Starting position   *2*   *3*

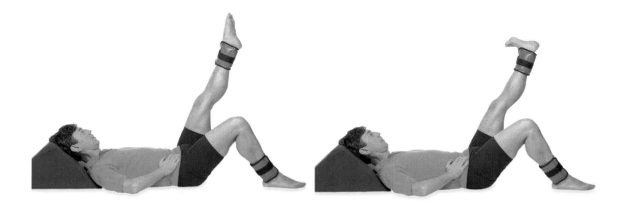

4 Breathe out. When the leg is straight, flex the foot and then, still zipped and hollowed, lower the leg, still turned out with foot flexed, almost to touch the floor. All the way down keep lengthening down the inside of the leg through the heel but keep the top of the thigh bone anchored into the hip socket. Do not allow the back to arch.

5 Breathe in and turn the leg into parallel from the hip. Softly point the foot.

6 Breathe out, still zipped and hollowed and bend the knee in again, turn it out from the hip and repeat the movement given in points 2 to 5.

7 Repeat ten times with each leg.

Watchpoints

- The most important aspect of this exercise is to keep the pelvis stable. Do not allow it to move from its neutral position. It should not tilt either to the north, the south, the east or the west!
- Think of keeping the length and width in the front of your pelvis to stop you from scrunching up.
- Do not flex the foot until the leg is fully straightened.
- Keep the leg in line with the hip. Do not allow it to go outside your body width.
- Keep the other foot flat on the floor but on an imagined chocolate cream eclair! No squashing it.

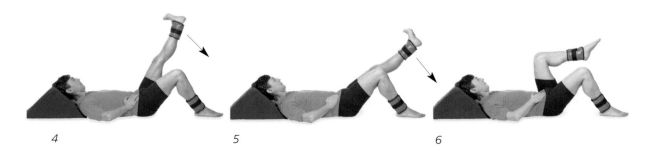

4   5   6

The Leg Weight Series: Battement

Aim

To teach stability in the pelvis while moving the legs. To strengthen the muscles which turn the leg out from the hip.

You need to be able to straighten your leg comfortably into the air for this exercise so your hamstrings should be a good length. Remember that the whole leg must be turned out from the hip joint itself.

Please take advice if you suffer from sciatica.

Starting Position

- Lie on your cushion, or in the Relaxation Position as for the previous exercise.
- Straighten one leg out in front of you, turned out from the hip. The foot softly pointed.
- The other leg remains bent, foot flat on the floor.

Action

1 Breathe in to prepare.
2 Breathe out, zip up and hollow.

3 Breathe in and raise the leg into the air, keeping it turned out and straight, keep your pelvis stable. Tailbone down.
4 Breathe out, still zipping and hollowing, flex the foot and slowly lower the leg almost to the floor. Lengthen down the inside of the leg through the heel.
5 Breathe in, softly point the foot and raise the leg again.
6 Repeat ten times on each leg. When you are confident with the movements, aim to raise the leg to a count of two and lower it to a count of four.

Watchpoints

1 Keep the pelvis steady and square.
2 Don't let the stomach muscles bulge.
3 The tailbone stays down!
4 The head of the thigh bone stays anchored into the hip socket.
5 Don't rely on the non working leg to stabilise you.

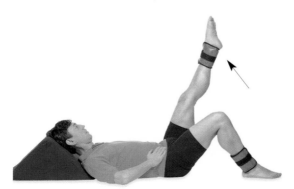
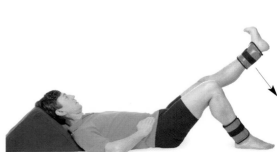

The Leg Weight Series: Circles

Aim

To strengthen the muscles round the hip. To learn fine control of the muscles round the hip. To stabilize the pelvis.

Please remember that we are after circles, not stars, squares or pentagons. Circles!

Starting Position

- Lie on your pillow, or in the Relaxation Position as for the previous two exercises.

Action

1 Breathe in to prepare.
2 Breathe out, zip up and hollow and bend and straighten one leg into the air above your hip. Hold the leg at an angle – see photo.
3 Breathing normally now, turn the leg out from your hip, keeping the pelvis stable. Flex the foot and slowly draw small circles in the air with the whole leg.
4 Draw ten circles in each direction with each leg.
5 Finish this series with a Pillow Squeeze (page 86) and/or a Relaxation (page 90).

Watchpoints

- Keep lengthening through the heel and the inside of the leg.
- Keep the leg anchored into the hip socket.
- Keep breathing.
- Keep hollowing to stabilize the pelvis.
- Keep the leg anchored into the hip joint, it should feel heavy.
- Keep the circles very small and very circular!!!
- Don't let the leg fall away from you.
- Don't rely on the other leg to stablise you – remember the chocolate eclair.

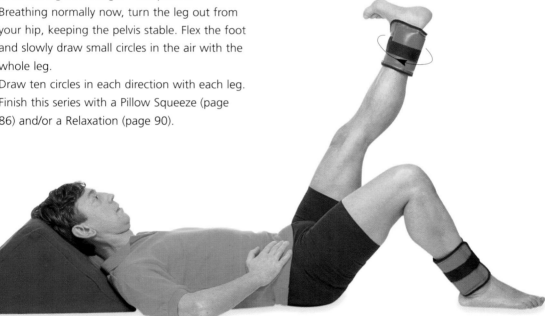

The Series Of Five – Feel The Powerhouse

These classical Pilates exercises done in succession will challenge both your strength and your stamina. Everything you have learnt as you have progressed through the levels will now be called upon. All Eight Principles are present in this advanced workout, none more so than centring. Joseph Pilates also referred to the girdle of strength as 'the power-house' – after doing this session we hope you will discover what he meant!

   Please note that this series does not constitute a balanced workout and that you will need to warm up before and wind down after performing it.

Warm up with:Spine Curls	p.45	
Hip Rolls	p.101	
Beach Ball Hamstring Stretch	p.123	
Roll Downs	p.68	
Chalk Circle	p.136	
Wind down with:The Diamond Press	p.110	
The Dart	p.70	
Side-lying Quadriceps and Hip Flexor Stretch	p.84	
The Pillow Squeeze	p.86	

1. The Single Leg Stretch

(See also page 106)

Starting Position
- Lie in the Relaxation Position.

Action
1 Breathe in to prepare.
2 Breathe out, zip up and hollow and fold your knees up onto your chest one at a time. The toes just touching – but not the heels. Keep your feet softly pointed. Place your hands on the outside of your calves.
3 Breathe in, check that your elbows are open to enable the chest to expand fully. Your shoulder blades are down into your back.
4 Breathe out, zip up and hollow, soften your breastbone and curl the upper body off the floor.
5 Breathe in and place the right hand on the outside of the right ankle, the left hand on the inside of the right knee.
6 Breathe out and, still zipping and hollowing, slowly stretch your left leg away in parallel, so that it is at an angle of 45° to the floor. The toes are softly pointed.
7 Breathe in wide and full, as you begin to bend the leg back onto your chest, bringing it back into your shoulder.
8 Change hands so that your left hand is on the outside of your left leg, your right hand on the inside of your left knee.

9 Breathe out and, still zipping and hollowing, stretch the right leg away in parallel. Do not take it too close to the floor.

10 Breathe in as the leg returns.

11 Repeat ten stretches on each leg, making sure that you have a strong centre throughout and that your shoulder blades stay down into your back, your elbows open.

Watchpoints

- Keep zipping and hollowing throughout and do not allow the back to arch, the pelvis stays neutral.
- Keep your neck released and the upper body open, shoulder blades down.
- Make sure you keep the length on both sides of your waist, do not allow one side to shorten.

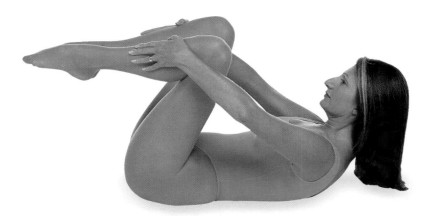

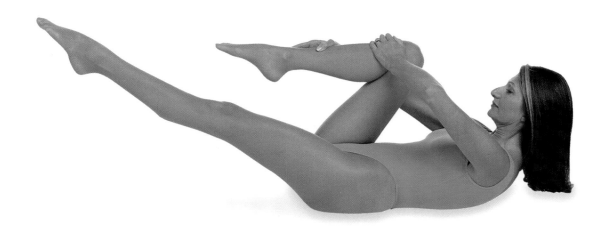

2. The Double Leg Stretch

(See also page 154)

Starting Position
- Lie with your knees bent, the knees are open from the hip. Your toes are just touching but your heels are apart. Have your hands resting on the outside of your knees.
- Your elbows are open, breastbone soft, shoulder blades down into your back.
- Gently roll your head from side to side to release the neck.

Action
1 Breathe out, zip up and hollow. These core muscles should stay engaged now throughout the exercise.
2 Breathe in and slowly curl your upper body up from the floor, gently tuck in the chin, at the same time straighten your legs so that they are turned out from the hips.
3 Flex the feet and lengthen up the inside of your legs to the heels. Squeeze the inner thighs together. Your fingers are lengthening away from you just below the knees on the outside of your thighs.
4 Breathe out, still zipped and hollowed and take your arms up in a wide sweep to the level of your ears, not behind. Keep the natural curve of the arms.
5 Breathe in as the arms circle back to return alongside the thighs again.
6 Breathe out as you slowly lower your head back down onto the floor, bending the knees so that they are back in the starting position.
7 Repeat ten times.

Watchpoints
- Do not allow the abdominals to bulge at all during the exercise, keep hollowing and keep lifting from the pelvic floor.
- Keep your neck long, the superficial muscles released.
- With the legs turned out and straight, make sure that you anchor the head of your thigh bones into the hips.
- Do not allow the legs to fall away.
- Do not take your arms behind the level of your ears.

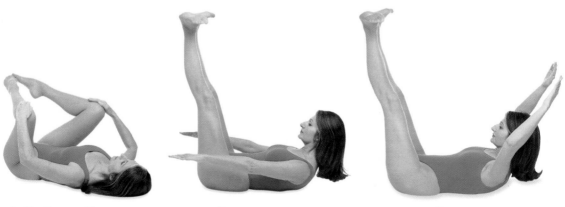

1. Starting position   2   3

3. Scissors

(See also page 160)

Starting Position

- Lie on the mat, zip up and hollow. Bring your knees, bent, onto your chest.
- Take hold of the right leg behind the thigh.

Action

1 Breathe in wide and full to prepare.
2 Breathe out, zip up and hollow (stay zipped and hollowed throughout now), curl the head and shoulders off the mat. Keep the breastbone soft.
3 Breathe in and straighten both legs up into the air, toes softly pointed. You are still holding the right leg behind the thigh.
4 Breathe out, lengthen the left leg towards the floor, stopping just above it.
5 Breathe in and raise the leg as straight as possible.
6 Breathe out and change arms and legs, lowering the right leg now.
7 Repeat ten times on each leg, aiming to cross over like scissors.

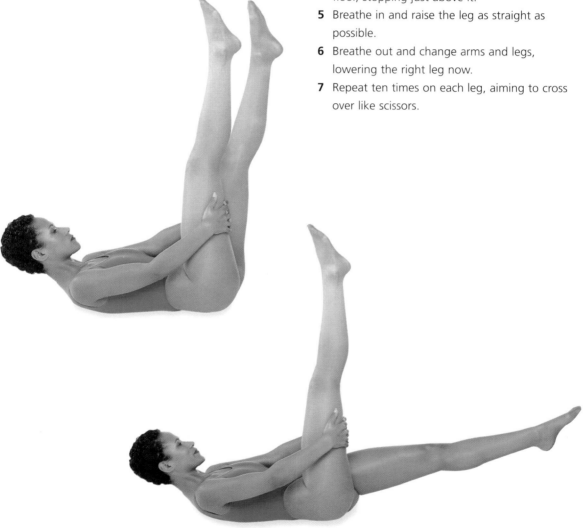

4. Double Straight Leg Lowers (Stages One and Two)

We have given you two versions here – the first is a preparation for the second more advanced version.

Stage One

Starting Position

• Lie in the Relaxation Position

Action

1 Breathe in wide and full to prepare.
2 Breathe out, zip up and hollow. Bend the knees up one at a time onto the chest.
3 Breathe in and stay zipped and hollowed throughout.
4 Breathe out and curl your head off the floor at the same time slowly straightening both legs into the air to an angle of 90°.
5 Breathe in and clasp behind both thighs (if you cannot reach, use a scarf).
6 Breathe out now and slowly lower both legs away from you without losing the neutral spinal and pelvic positions and without allowing your abdominals to bulge. Do not lower the legs too far.
7 Breathe in as you slowly raise the legs to 90° again.
8 Repeat eight times.

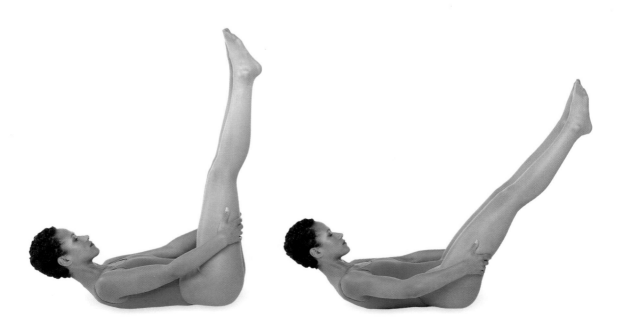

Stage Two

Starting Position
- Lie in the Relaxation Position but have your hands gently clasped behind your head, elbows just in front of your ears.

Action
1 Breathe in to prepare.
2 Breathe out, zip up and hollow (stay zipped and hollowed throughout the exercise) and bend the knees up one at a time.
3 Breathe in and slowly curl the head off the floor, straightening both legs up to an angle of 90°. Make this movement slow and controlled.
4 Breathe out and hold the position.
5 Breathe in and slowly lower both legs away from you just a little (see below). Your pelvis must stay neutral, your abdominals hollow.
6 Breathe out and raise the legs again.
7 Repeat this action, breathing in as you lower, out as you raise the legs up, ten times. The lower you take the legs the harder the challenge. You have been warned!

Watchpoints
- At no time should you allow your back to arch, you must stay neutral. To do this you must use your abdominals.
- Check that you are not pulling on your neck, you should have no tension there, your neck should be released, your breastbone soft.

Moving on ...

Try a different breathing pattern, with a double action for each breath in and out. Breathing in to lower the legs down and up and breathing out to lower the legs down and up

Variation
Try having the legs in a turned out position.

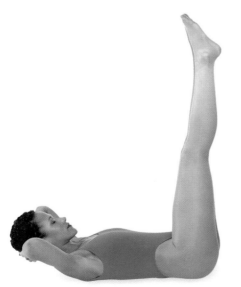
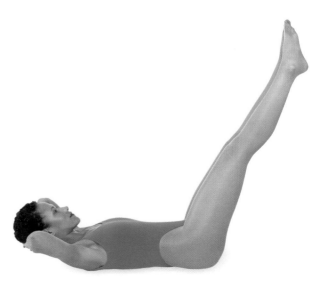

5. Oblique Single Leg Stretch (Criss Cross)

(See also page 163)

Starting Position

- Lie on your back, draw your knees up onto your chest, the toes just touching – but not the heels. Keep your feet softly pointed.
- Clasp your hands behind your head. The elbows stay open.

Action

1 Breathe in wide and full to prepare.
2 Breathe out, zip up and hollow as you curl up, softening the breastbone and taking the right shoulder in the direction of your left knee. The upper body stays open, the elbows in line. At the same time straighten the right leg, extending it in parallel at an angle of about 45° to the floor.
3 Breathe out, still zipped and hollowed and curl the left shoulder towards the right bent knee, extending the left leg away.
4 Repeat ten times to each side.

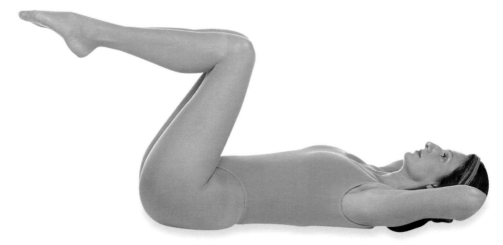

Starting position

Watchpoints

- Make sure that the shoulder, not the elbow, comes across towards the bent knee.
- Keep the elbows in line, do not allow them to come forward – it is your shoulder that is directed towards the knee. In this way, the upper body stays open.
- Stay neutral please.

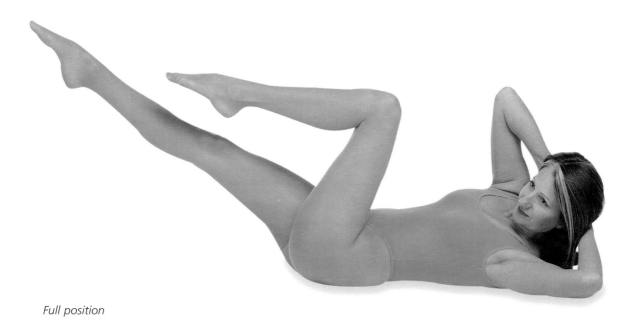

Full position

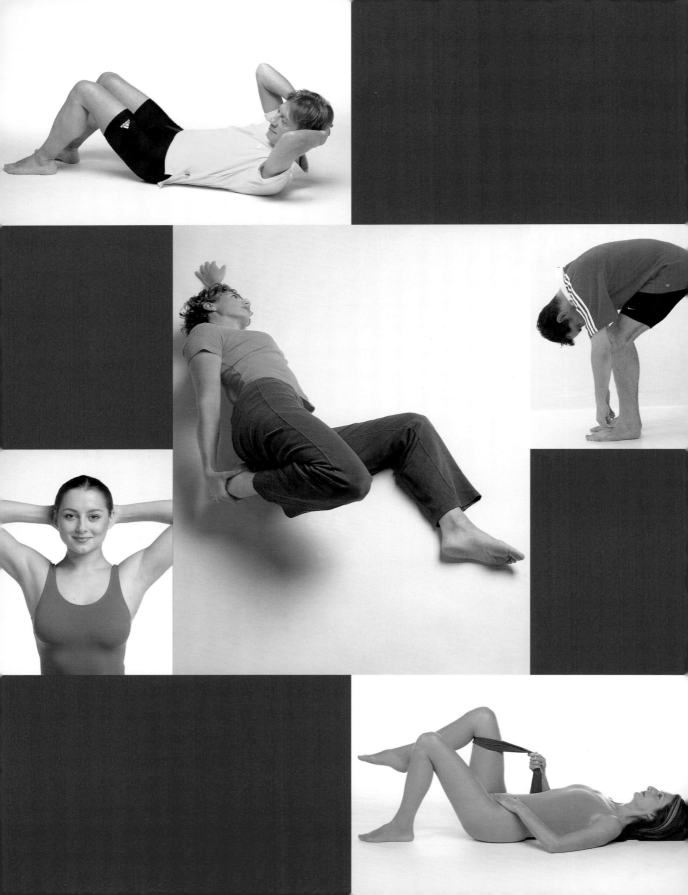

Body Control Pilates
at Work

We have already seen how the input our nervous system receives has a direct influence on how we move. If we spend eight hours a day sitting, standing or repeating certain movements, it will invariably affect our movement patterns. Working conditions play a large role in determining our postural alignment. Of course, hereditary factors, illness, trauma, injury and so on contribute to our postural type as well, but holding sustained positions or performing repetitive movements again and again will affect the way we move.

In the following chapters, we have studied some of the more common professions and the problems which they may engender. With this in mind, we have recommended exercise routines that should be used in conjunction with the remedial programmes designed to correct your postural type. Practised regularly, the exercises will help prevent problems occurring.

Sedentary Workers

Jobs which involve sitting at a desk all day are likely to have a detrimental effect on our health unless we counter the lack of movement with corrective exercise.

Well-designed work stations go a long way to helping the problem but the bottom line is that you are still glued to the desk for hours on end, often sitting with the spine rotating regularly one way. Much will depend on how you sit, far too many of us slouch which causes postural strain.

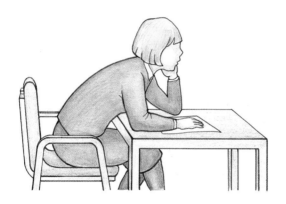

Sitting incorrectly causes postural strain

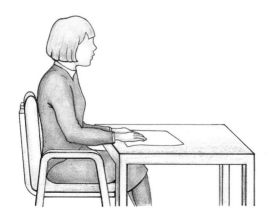

The end result of sitting badly all day will probably be the following:

- Weak transversus abdominis
- Tight upper rectus abdominis
- Tight dominant hip flexors
- Rounded thoracic spine
- Tight pectorals, especially if you work at a computer
- Medially (inwardly) rotated shoulder blades
- Tight levator scapulae (elevating the shoulder blades)
- Tight upper trapezius
- Head poking forward leading to weak deep neck flexors and tight neck extensors
- Tight adductors and medial rotators of the hip especially if you sit cross-legged
- Weak gluteals
- A rotated, twisted spine

It is also possible that you may be prone to CPRS 1 and 2, which stands for Complex Pain Related Syndrome (World Health Organization definition) commonly known as repetitive strain injury or elbow ache to the rest of us! This is a controversial issue among medical professionals because, as with any problem of this nature, there are many factors involved. It seems that the nervous system can become oversensitive. It is not within the scope of this book to delve any further, however, we can recommend exercises that will help deter the onset of these conditions. If you are already suffering from such a problem you will need to consult your specialist.

First, let's get you sitting better at work.

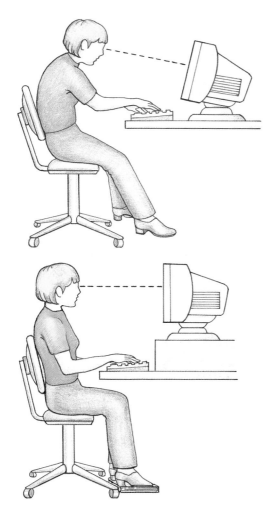

Zip up and hollow while sitting correctly	p.34	
Ankle Circles sitting at your desk	p.44	
Side Reaches Sitting and Standing	p.64	
The Cossack	p.62	
Tricep Stretch	p.128	
The Dumb Waiter	p.56	
The Corkscrew	p.96	
Up and Down with a Tennis Ball	p.88	
Standing Quadriceps Stretch	p.134	
Roll Downs against the wall, or free-standing	p.68	

You may need a lumbar roll or wedge to help you maintain the natural curves of the spine. Keep an eye out for a new invention – a rubber air-filled cushion which you sit on to help you maintain good posture. If possible invest in a chair specifically tailored to your needs (see addresses in the back of the book).Now you are sitting comfortably, we need to get you up and moving again. During your coffee, lunch and tea breaks instead of nipping outside for a ciggie break, try the following exercises which can easily be done, without undue embarrassment, in the office environment.

And at the end of the day take just a few moments to 'iron out the body'. Follow your recommended programme according to your specific postural type (pages 14–18) adding the following exercises:

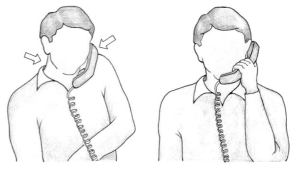

Avoid cradling the phone in your neck. Keep both shoulder blades down, neck released as if using a hands free phone.

Relaxation Position	p.28		Side Reaches	p.64	
The Starfish	p.42		Roll Downs	p.68	
Knee Stirs	p.43		Waist Twists with a Pole (avoid if you have CPRS 1 or 2)	p.63	
Shoulder Drops	p.48		Pole Raises	p.60	
Neck Rolls	p.50		The Diamond Press	p.110	
Spine Curls	p.45		The Dart	p.70	
Hip Flexor Stretch	p.47		The Star	p.114	
Side Rolls	p.54		Rest Position	p.73	
Hamstring Stretch	p.82		Side-lying Quadriceps and Hip Flexor Stretch	p.84	
Curl Ups	p.78		Arm Openings or Chalk Circle	p.52 or p.136	
Oblique Curl Ups	p.79				

'Pilates has changed my life. I've gone from needing weekly visits to the osteopath, to having complete confidence in my own body. Before Pilates classes with Lynne, I was afraid to do even the most gentle of daily tasks in case I put my back out. Now my whole posture has changed. I am stronger, leaner and fitter than I've ever been. I feel and look great. And I haven't seen the osteopath for months.'

Shelley Sishton, Marketing Consultant

The Medical Profession

We've divided the medical profession into two groups: those who tend to be on their feet all day bending over patients, such as doctors, dentists, opticians and surgeons (Group One); and nurses who combine the above with heavy lifting (Group Two).

The majority of both groups work long, unsociable shifts and suffer from high stress levels, so we've added a few extra relaxing exercises.

Add the following exercises to those recommended for your specific postural type (pages 14–18).

Group One

Relaxation Position	p.28	
Spine Curls	p.45	
Hip Flexor Stretch	p.47	
Curl Ups	p.78	
Oblique Curl Ups	p.79	
Side Rolls	p.54	
Side-lying Quadriceps Stretch and Hip Flexor Stretch	p.84	
Hamstring Stretch	p.82	
The Diamond Press	p.110	
The Dart	p.70	

The Star	p.114	
Rest Position (unless you have knee problems)	p.73	
Roll Downs	p.68	
The Corkscrew	p.96	
The Dumb Waiter	p.56	
Arm Openings	p.52	
Relaxation Position	p.28	

Group Two

Stability while lifting is crucial here, as are strong thigh muscles so that you may bend the knees as you lift.

Relaxation Position	p.28	
Spine Curls	p.45	
Pelvic Stability	p.38	
Curl Ups (replace with Single Leg Stretch/Double Leg Stretch when you are strong enough)	p.78 (p.106, p.108)	
Oblique Curl Ups	p.79	
Hip Flexor Stretch	p.47	

Side Rolls	p.54	
Sliding Down the Wall	p.66	
Up and Down with a Tennis Ball	p.88	
Roll Downs	p.68	
The Diamond Press or The Dart	p.110 or p.70	
Table Top	p.118	

Rest Position	p.73	
Ankle Circles on the Wall	p.133	
Cherry Picking	p.189	
Wide Leg Stretch Against a Wall (see Adductor Stretch)	p.80	
Passé Développés	p.170	
Arm Openings	p.52	

'It is wonderful to have found a method of exercise to . . . help us uncoil, to lengthen, to "iron us out" . . . I know that many of my patients would benefit enormously from these exercises.'

Richard Husband, MB, Ch.B., DRCOG

Standing Professions

This includes shop assistants, hairdressers, police officers, schoolteachers, exercise instructors, physiotherapists, waitresses, bus conductors.

Do you stand for your living? The above and hosts of other professions do and may suffer from tired aching legs, spinal compression, low back ache, varicose veins, sore feet and dropped arches to name but a few of the more glamorous perks of the trade!

Add the following exercises to those recommended for your postural type on pages 14–18.

Spine Curls	p.45	
Ankle Circles on the Wall	p.133	
Wide Leg Stretch Against a Wall	p.81	
Foot Exercises (see also opposite)	pp.74-5	
The Diamond Press	p.110	
The Dart	p.70	
Rest Position	p.73	
Side-lying Quadriceps and Hip Flexor Stretch	p.84	
Arm Openings	p.52	

Add the following exercise to your programme. It works the calf pump which will help improve the circulation and lymphatic drainage in your legs.

Exercise: Cherry Picking

Starting Position

- Lie on your back in the Relaxation Position.
- Bend one knee up and take hold of it just behind the knee, with your thumbs coming round in front of the knee – this is so that you can feel if your leg is moving.
- Soften your elbows and open your chest.

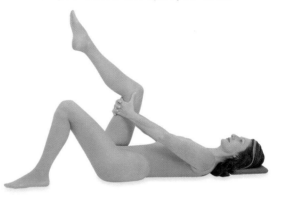

Action

1 Keeping your heel still and in line with your knees and hips, flex the foot towards your face, then flex the toes towards your face and spread them as wide as possible.

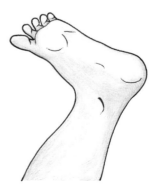

2 Keeping them flexed, push through the ball of your foot as you straighten the foot, keeping the heel still.

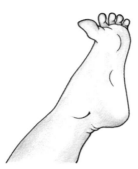

3 Now imagine that a cherry tree is there – pick a cherry from it by clasping it with the toes.

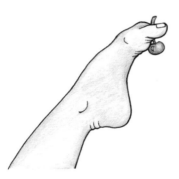

4 Keeping the prized cherry firmly clasped in your toes, flex the foot back towards your face.
5 Drop the cherry into an imaginary basket and let go of the foot.
6 Collect five cherries with each foot!

Exercise: Foot Massage

If your feet ache after standing all day you might also like to try a foot massage. Do not do this if your foot is injured in any way.

Starting Position

- Wash your feet with some warm water in order to increase the circulation and soften the skin. Sit comfortably in your favourite chair with plenty of cushions to support your back.
- Depending on the range of movement in your hip joint:
- Sit cross-legged and place one foot on the opposite thigh – don't worry if you cannot do this, only a few people are able to while leaving the rest of the body relaxed.
- Or draw one leg up with the knee towards your chest, keeping the leg in parallel. This way you can easily reach the back of the foot and the sole with the fingers.
- Or work with a partner, who sits on the floor in front of you while supporting your knee with cushions.

Action

1 Stroke the whole of the foot with a flat, relaxed hand, not forgetting to include the ankles. You might want to use a little moisturizing lotion to glide more easily. When working with a partner, use a firm but soft touch to help them relax and at the same time reassure them.
2 Circle one toe at a time gently in its socket.
3 Pinch the skin between the toes with the thumb and the index finger.
4 With two to three fingers, circle all over the foot – avoid the ankles if you or your partner are pregnant or are trying to conceive.
5 Press with your thumbs on the bottom of your foot (this might be a little painful, especially round the instep of your foot). You should do whatever feels good, so, when you are working with a partner, always ask for their comments and guidance.

Flying High

Whether you are pilot, cabin crew or passenger, air travel will take its toll on your body. Let's look at each in turn:

We have devised and tested a pre-flight routine and one which can and should be done in mid-air. In addition, we have given each group specific after-flight exercises to rebalance the body.

Once in the air everyone will have problems from the increase in pressure, restricted movement and circulation, dehydration and jet lag. The following will help:

Before the Flight

Relaxation Position with Breathing and Stabilization	p.37	
Spine Curls	p.45	
Side Rolls	p.54	
Hamstring Stretch	p.82	
Windmill Arms	p.102	
Curl Ups	p.78	
Oblique Curl Ups	p.79	
Single Leg Stretch	p.106	
Pole Raises	p.60	
Side Reaches Standing	p.64	

The Dart	p.70	
Rest Position	p.73	

In the Air

Roll Downs	p.68	
Advanced Warm Up: Walking on the Spot	p.140	
Sliding Down the Wall (or the outside of the loo door)	p.66	
Standing Quadriceps Stretch	p.134	
Triceps Stretch	p.128	
The Dumb Waiter	p.56	
The Corkscrew	p.96	
Standing on One Leg	p.94	
The Cossack	p.62	
Side Reaches	p.64	
Foot exercises which can be done sitting and will help reduce swelling: Ankle Circles, Point and Flex	p.74, p.44, p.76	
Mexican Wave	p.75	

In the Cockpit

In many ways you can compare a pilot to a driver, sitting for long periods of time in a confined space with very few opportunities to stretch the legs, with irregular sleeping patterns and high stress levels. We've put together some simple stretches and strengthening exercises that will be perfect to do either before or after a flight:

Spine Curls	p.45	
Hip Flexor Stretch	p.47	
Hamstring Stretch	p.82	
Side Rolls	p.54	
The Diamond Press	p.110	
The Dart	p.70	
The Rest Position	p.73	
Adductor Stretch	p.80	
Side Reaches Standing	p.64	
Side-lying Quadriceps and Hip Flexor Stretch	p.84	
Roll Downs	p.68	
Arm Openings or Chalk Circle	p.52 or p.136	

The Cabin Crew

The cabin crew have a different set of problems to the flight crew. They are concerned with hospitality and the comfort and care of the passengers. This involves being on their feet non-stop and repeated bending and twisting as they reach to pass the person in seat 57A his lunch! Those food trolleys require careful manoeuvring and pushing, plus helping to lift hand luggage into the overhead lockers – and how many of us are over our limit? All these actions require very strong abdominals and good stability plus flexibility. Mind you, with air rage becoming increasingly common perhaps we should add some more physical skills to the list of requirements!

After the flight

Starfish	p.42	
Ankle Circles on the Wall	p.133	
Hip Rolls	p.101	
Shoulder Drops	p.48	
Adductor Stretch	p.80	
Beach Ball Hamstring Stretch	p.123	
Threading a Needle	p.77	
Single Heel Kicks	p.112	
The Dart	p.70	

The Diamond Press	p.110	
Rest Position	p.73	
Table Top with Sliding Legs	p.119	
Chalk Circle	p.136	

On Arrival

Long-haul flights are a nightmare if you suffer from back problems and can be a nightmare even if you do not! However, you can keep yourself mobile in the air by following the In the Air routine given above – these can all be done on an aeroplane, providing the seat belt sign isn't on! You will not believe how much better you'll feel when you arrive at your destination and, to help you further after you arrive, try:

Relaxation Position	p.28	
Spine Curls	p.45	
Hip Flexor Stretch	p.47	

Hamstring Stretch	p.82	
Curl Ups	p.78	
Side Rolls	p.54	
Side-lying Quadriceps and Hip Flexor Stretch	p.84	
The Corkscrew	p.96	
Side Reach	p.64	
Pole Raises	p.60	
Roll Downs	p.68	
The Diamond Press	p.110	
Rest Position	p.73	
Arm Openings or Chalk Circle	p.52 or p.136	

One other tip, if you do have a stopover, always use the opportunity to walk briskly round the airport to wake everything up!

'Like so many people, my work entails remaining seated for long periods . . . This frequently leads to muscular aches and pains, and an associated loss of suppleness. Pilates enables me to exercise virtually anywhere, at any time – even in my seat. When I get to my hotel, the full range of Pilates exercises are easily completed in the privacy of my own room . . . I recommend Body Control Pilates to all my colleagues and anyone else who wants to maximize their body's "potential."

Sean Volrath, Boeing 747 *Classic* Pilot

Manual Workers

If your job involves a lot of manual labour it will naturally involve a lot of movement. Movement is good but unfortunately these jobs often involve heavy lifting and twisting and if you are not stable you may have problems. Remember we need the right muscles to be working in the right way.

Your conditioning programme should involve developing your deep postural muscles and increasing your awareness of moving correctly. Add the following exercises to those recommended for your postural type:

The Starfish	p.42	
Spine Curls	p.45	
Hip Flexor Stretch	p.47	
Pelvic Stability	p.38	
Side Rolls	p.54	
Beach Ball Hamstrings	p.123	

Curl Ups	p.78	
Oblique Curl Ups	p.79	
The Hundred	p.120	
The Corkscrew	p.96	
Roll Downs	p.68	
Side Reaches	p.64	
Pole Raises	p.60	
The Dart	p.70	
Table Top (adding arm and leg movements)	p.118	
Single Heel Kicks	p.112	
Rest Position	p.73	
Chalk Circle	p.136	

Driving for a Living

Do you drive for a living? Wether you are a long-haul truck driver or a sales rep, or a Formula One driver – you will be sitting trapped in one position which places enormous strain on your back.

Long-distance drivers should add the following exercises to those recommended for their postural type:

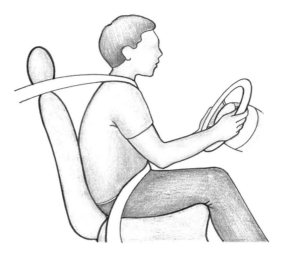

Poor posture while driving will strain your back

The Starfish	p.42	
Spine Curls	p.45	
Hip Flexor Stretch	p.47	
Neck Rolls	p.50	
Nose Spirals	p.264	
Nodding Dog	p.264	
Curl Ups	p.78	
Oblique Curl Ups	p.79	
Side Rolls	p.54	
Knee Stirs	p.43	
Shoulder Drops	p.48	
Side-lying Quadriceps and Hip Flexor Stretch	p.84	

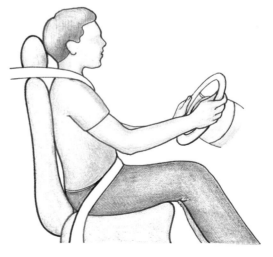

Try to keep lengthening up and maintain the natural curves of the spine

The Diamond Press	p.110	
The Dart	p.70	
The Star	p.114	
Rest Position	p.73	
Roll Downs	p.68	

Side Reaches	p.64	
Finger Exercises	p.229	
Foot Exercises	p.74	
Arm Openings	p.52	

'. . . I shall certainly be recommending this book to my patients as a complement to what they have learnt in the treatment room . . . I look forward to Pilates teaching becoming more common, so that I can safely refer my patients to an exercise class confident that they will not re-injure themselves.'

Physiotherapy Magazine, UK
(reviewing *Body Control: The Pilates Way*)

'Some patients referred to Pilates teachers never need further regular treatment, and many only begin to maintain improvement once they take up Pilates.'

Piers Chandler, DO
Osteopath

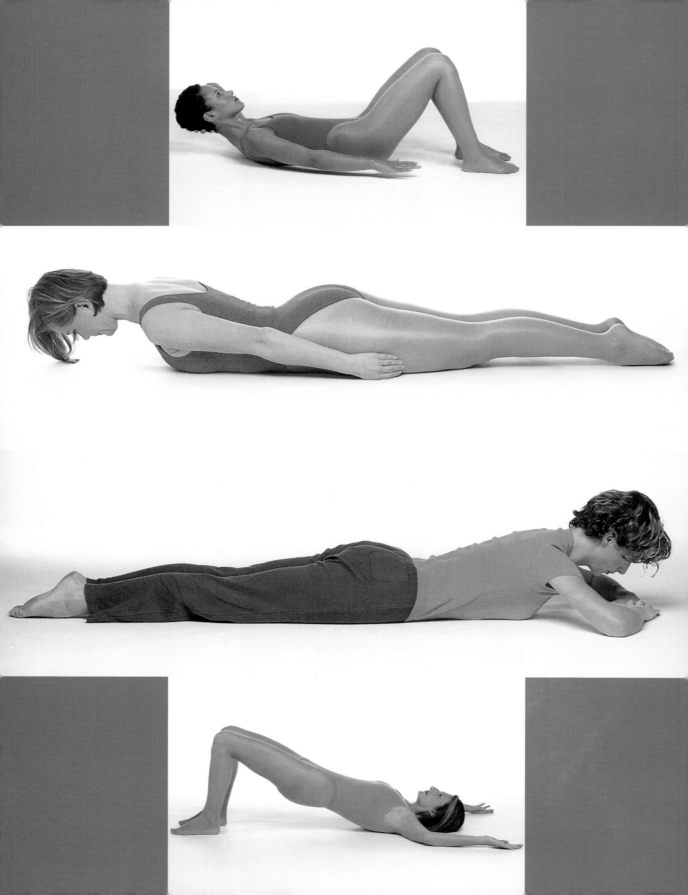

Body Control Pilates
at Work
at Play

Body Control Pilates is an ideal exercise system for sports people. It establishes a strong postural base from which they can develop their sporting technique more safely and efficiently. If only they started it before rather than after they get injured!

Dr Charlotte Cowie
MBBS, D Sport Med., DM-S Med., MRO

Swimming is a very technique-dependent sport. Incorrect methods will lead to muscle fatigue and/or muscle imbalances, which lead to altered performance.

Body Control Pilates is now being utilized by swimmers to establish correct method and muscle conditioning to enhance techniques which are specific to the demands of their stroke, and so improve their performance.

Paul Massey BA MCSP SRP
Head Physiotherapist Great Britain Swimming Team. British Olympic team member 1992 and 1996. Team staff to Great Britain Athletic team. National Coaching Foundation Senior Tutor.

The following pages are dedicated to sport. The advice given is aimed mainly at the professional or semi-professional, however, the enthusiastic amateur will benefit equally from these exercises.

Have you noticed how, alongside the rapid growth in the number of fitness and sports centres, there has been an equivalent growth in the number of sports injury clinics? Why should this be so when sport increases fitness and health?

At amateur level there is the problem of people playing a game for which they are not fit. Middle-aged, born-again footballers, for example, taking up the game after years of absence and without proper training who don't go regularly to training sessions and whose bodies are neither flexible nor strong enough to cope with the rigours of the game.

Another problem lies with the nature of the sport itself. Many sports are unilateral, in other words they develop one side of the body or one set of muscles only. Take golf for example – you repeatedly bend over the ball, rotating the spine and hitting the ball one way only. This places enormous, repetitive strain on the lumbar spine. Part of the difficulty would be resolved if you played the first nine holes right-handed and the back nine left-handed, but even then you would still be using the same sets of muscles while totally ignoring others. You are also still bent over the ball! Training techniques which focus on strengthening the muscles you need to be able to hit the ball further can merely add to the problem. These muscles are already strong enough

and you should really be more concerned with the muscles which are ignored when playing a round, as their relative weakness will unbalance the body and may lead to an increased risk of injury.

Each sport requires its players to have certain motor patterns, this is the skill they need to play their sport well, and heaven help us if we try to alter the way a top golfer swings, a tennis player serves or a cricketer bowls. However, a few well-designed exercises added to a regular training routine will ensure that the body becomes more balanced and the movement patterns remain normal. The end result will be fewer injuries, faster recuperation from trauma injury, and a better performance all round as the body becomes more efficient. By establishing sound muscle recruitment patterns a competitor will play better and longer, and hopefully be able to enjoy post-sport years free from pain. We have worked with several top sportsmen who now realize that if they had known about this approach earlier, their careers at the highest level might have been extended by several years.

So, in the following chapters we have studied the most common problems associated with the most popular sports and we've chosen a few extra exercises which should be added to those recommended for each postural type. Once thee basics are mastered and stability achieved it is vital that we challenge that stability in as many ways as possible. The programmes recommended are not designed to replace traditional training regimes but to supplement them.

Football

With many Premier League footballers earning in excess of one million pounds a year, it is no surprise that injuries are perhaps the biggest headache for managers and players alike. Many of the injuries sustained on the football pitch are unavoidable, resulting from the inherently physical nature of the game, but many injuries which can lay players off for several weeks are certainly avoidable if only footballers were to pay more attention to the balance of their muscles. Fortunately many of the physiotherapists attached to football clubs and academies are now using Pilates to help prevent injuries.

'I see the *Body Control Pilates* method, with a focus on muscle balance, as an important aspect in the prevention of injury.'

Alan Hodson MA, MCSP, SRP
Head of Sports Medicine,
The English Football Association

Some of the most common football injuries include: groin injuries, hamstring strains, cruciate ligament injuries, ankle injuries, trauma injuries from tackles and back problems, especially disc-related ones exacerbated by the way in which players kick the ball from their back, not their hip.

Much of the problem lies with muscle imbalance in the body. The nature of the game means that many footballers have the following imbalances:

- Strong, overworked quadriceps
- Strong, tight hamstrings
- Shortened anterior ankle muscles e.g. tibialis anterior
- Tight calf muscles

- Tight hip flexors
- Overworked back extensors (erector spinae)
- Weak gluteals
- Weak transversus abdominis
- Weak multifidus

The end result is a body with poor trunk and pelvic stability and very poor flexibility. On top of this almost every footballer – even at the highest level – favours one leg or one side, so you also have a unilateral imbalance. No wonder they are often on the bench!

As a footballer, add the following exercises to the recommended programme for your postural type:

Roll Downs	p.68	
Spine Curls	p.45	
Hip Flexor Stretch	p.47	
Hamstring Stretch	p.82	
Side Rolls	p.54	
Side-lying Quadriceps Stretch (if no knee injuries)	p.84	
Curl Ups with Arm Action	p.104	
Single Leg Stretch or The Hundred or Double Leg Stretch	p.106 or p.120 or p.108	

Oblique Curl Ups	p.79		Rest Position	p.73	
The Dart	p.70		Passé Développés series (for strengthening gluteus medius)	p.170	
Table Top with Sliding Legs	p.119		Standing on one Leg	p.94	

'The last few years have seen an acceptance that good core stability assessment and exercise prescription are essential considerations in the treatment of any spinal (and, in many cases, peripheral) mechanical complaints and in the management of injury prevention of those involved in sport.

However, the … approach developed by Joseph Pilates was addressing many aspects of core stabilty, and a great deal more besides, over 80 years ago!

The fact that his system has evolved into what we now know as Body Control Pilates is a testament to both the vision and talent of Joseph Pilates and those, like Lynne Robinson, who have promoted his work and refined it into something which is rapidly becoming the osteopath's first-choice recommendation to patients recovering from almost any injury.

The knowledge base and level of continued personal development of those involved in the Body Control Pilates Association are of a standard that many other therapy approaches could do well to emulate. I would honestly say that, once you've seen (and experienced) how powerful Body Control Pilates can be, you'll wish you had taken it up years ago!'

Jonathan Betser DO
Chairman of the UK Osteopathic Sports Care Association

Rugby

Visualize the pre-match line up at Twickenham, and the contrast in physiques as you pass along the line – the light nippy winger, the squat prop forward, the heavy yet mobile back row forward.

Different positions need different physiques, and engender different muscle imbalances and greater susceptibility to certain types of injuries: prop forwards get neck and shoulder problems – no wonder with the total weight of two packs (often exceeding 1.5 tonnes) bearing down on them in the scrum; wingers get tackled at high speed by larger, weightier opponents. Generally speaking, rugby players have strength but not flexibility. The answer, however, does not lie simply in stretching tight muscles but in altering movement patterns so that the tight muscles can release and stay at their optimal length. In rugby, much of the game is played in a semi-crouching, forward-leaning position – it's no wonder rugby players have back pain.

As a contact sport, rugby involves a lot of trauma injuries, alongside the more frequent injuries such as groin strains, neck injuries, whiplash, back and rib injuries.

Common problems among players are:

- Over-developed shoulder and neck muscles, usually in front-row forwards
- Especially tight upper trapezius to support the neck
- Overworking levator scapulae
- Poor pelvic stability due to weak transversus abdominis, pelvic floor and multifidus
- Tight dominating adductors
- Weak gluteals
- Tight hip flexors
- Overworked hamstrings
- Arched, tight lower backs
- Overdeveloped pectorals

To counter much of this, add the following exercises to the recommended postural programme:

Spine Curls	p.45	
Hip Flexor Stretch	p.47	
Pelvic Stability	p.38	
Side Rolls (Hip Rolls)	p.54 (p.101)	
Curl Ups	p.78	
Oblique Curl Ups	p.79	
Hamstring Stretch	p.82	
Pole Raises	p.60	
Standing on One Leg	p.94	
The Dumb Waiter	p.56	
Side Reaches	p.64	
The Corkscrew	p.96	
Roll Downs	p.68	

Side-lying Quadriceps and Hip Flexor Stretch	p.84	
The Dart	p.70	
The Star	p.114	
Table Top (adding arms and legs)	p.119	

Passé Développés	p.170	
Rest Position	p.73	
Arm Openings	p.52	

Cricket

'After persistent back problems earlier in the year I found Pilates exercises, in conjunction with sound orthopaedic advice, to have been enormously beneficial. The exercises are now a daily routine for me and I am sure that they are, in a large way responsible for me being able to continue my cricketing career.'

Mike Atherton
(England cricketer)

At the 1998 Sporting Back Conference of the British Institute for Musculoskeletal Medicine and the Society of Orthopaedic Medicine, Dr Philip Bell, the England cricket team doctor, pointed out that almost all fast bowlers over the age of eighteen years of age – with the notable exception of the West Indians, which he attributed to their natural flexibility – suffer from lumbar spine problems, particularly spondylolithesis or stress fractures. A lot of the young talent in cricket will never make it through to the highest level because of these injuries.

This alarming fact comes as no surprise when you watch a fast bowler's action and delivery, with its combined rotation, flexion and extension of the spine at speed and with the full weight of their own body placing enormous repetitive stress on the same part of the lumbar spine.

And that's just the bowlers. Batting involves flexion and rotation, wicket keepers are in an especially difficult position as they squat behind the stumps with their heads thrown back and arms extended, slip fielders adopt a similar though less extreme position, fielders in the cover or boundary positions collect and throw the ball in one twisting motion placing extreme pressure on their back, shoulders and arms.

Common cricketing injuries include stress fractures of the lumbar spine, shoulder problems, neck problems, stress fractures of the feet. Problems include:

- unstable pelvis
- unstable lumbar spine
- lack of scapular stability

Cricketers should add the following exercises to their recommended postural programme:

Four Point Kneeling	p.35	
The Starfish	p.42	
Pelvic Stability	p.38	
Spine Curls	p.45	
Hip Flexor Stretch	p.47	
Hamstring Stretch	p.82	
Side Rolls (when stable)	p.54	
Pole Raises	p.60	
The Corkscrew	p.96	
The Dumb Waiter	p.56	

The Dart	p.70	
The Diamond Press	p.110	
Table Top	p.118	

Rest Position	p.73	
Side-lying Quadriceps and Hip Flexor Stretch	p.84	
Arm Openings or Chalk Circle	p.52 or p.136	

Racquet Sports

'Pilates is the ideal workout, relaxing, soothing, mentally and physically challenging with the aggressive impact on the body. When I have an ailment I head straight for the Pilates studio. It has kept me in one piece for years.'

Pat Cash

(former Wimbledon Singles Tennis Champion)

Pat Cash, a former Wimbledon tennis champion, was one of the first sportsmen to feel the benefit of a Pilates programme. Super fit and having tried many different fitness techniques which put a lot of strain on his body, he had ignored his deep stabilizing muscles. Like many sports, tennis is asymmetrical and this had resulted in Pat developing a serious muscle imbalance problem which led to a disc injury. Following surgery, which left him, in his own words, 'as stiff as a board', his physiotherapist introduced him to Pilates and, within a remarkably short period of time, he was back playing top-level tennis again.

Playing a game of tennis involves frequent twisting, turning and changing direction at speed. The tennis serve itself involves rotation with flexion and speed, placing stress on the lumbar spine and shoulder. Good playing technique can go a long way to helping prevent injury – for example if a player uses his whole body rather than just his shoulder muscles to serve he can avoid problems and a good, fluent forehand or backhand stroke will help prevent tennis or badminton elbow.

Common injuries include shoulder joint impingement problems, tight medial rotators of the shoulders, knee injuries, Achilles tendonitis, lumbar spine injuries and neck injuries.

The problems?

- Lumbar instability
- Pelvic instability
- Overworked neck extensors
- Overworked levator scapulae
- Tight pectorals and anterior deltoids leading to rounded shoulders
- Tight latissimus dorsi
- The thoracic spine held in flexion
- Overworked forearms (especially if you constantly spin the ball which means you are continually rotating the wrist and elbow)

Add the following exercises to those recommended for your postural type:

Roll Downs	p.68	
Spine Curls	p.45	
Neck Rolls	p.50	
Shoulder Drops	p.48	
Hamstring Stretch	p.82	
Side-lying Quadriceps and Hip Flexor Stretch	p.84	
Oblique Curl Ups or Oblique Single Leg Stretch	p.79 (or p.180)	
Single Leg Stretch	p.106	
The Hundred	p.120	

Double Leg Stretch	p.108		Rest Position	p.73	
Windmill Arms	p.102		Wrist Worker	p.255	
The Diamond Press	p.110		The Corkscrew	p.96	
The Dart	p.70		Pole Raisers	p.60	
Threading a Needle	p.77		Arm Openings or Chalk Circle	p.52 or p.136	

Golf

It is easy to appreciate why so many golfers have back problems, just lifting the golf bag out of the car boot, hitching it onto your shoulder and carrying it to the first tee puts an enormous strain on your back – and you haven't even hit the ball yet!

Like so many other sports golf is asymmetrical, in that it totally unbalances the body. Just think about it . . . you play eighteen holes over three or four hours, during which time you are constantly bending over the ball and repeatedly twisting your body in the same way. You are therefore using the same muscles and reinforcing the same bent over posture again and again. As a result, these muscles are overused while their counterparts are ignored, leaving whole groups of muscles unused.

Professional golfers are more prone to overuse injuries as a result of the sheer number of times that they swing a club. The shoulders, neck, hips and feet are all vulnerable, but it is the spine which takes the greatest toll. Medical scans have shown that professional right-handed golfers have above average damage on their right sides, where the twist from the swing has its devastating effect, leaving them prone to low back problems as serious as herniated discs. Although amateur golfers do not play as frequently as professionals, they are usually far from fit when they go out on the golf course and can suffer similar injuries.

Common injuries include lumbar spine injury, hip problems and shoulder and neck injuries.

Common muscle imbalances include:

- Dominating back extensors (erector spinae)
- Lack of lumbar and pelvic stability
- Tight pectorals and anterior deltoids leading to rounded shoulders
- Weak lower trapezius and serratus anterior
- Thoracic spine held in flexion
- Overworked neck extensors
- Overworked forearms leading to problems with the grip

We have given two sets of additional exercises here, the first can be done on the golf course as a warm up, the second is for after the game to rebalance the body.

Pre-round warm up

Standing with preparation breathing, lengthening and centring	p.56	
Roll Downs	p.68	
Waist Twist using a wood	p.62	
Side Reaches	p.64	
Pole Raises using a club	p.60	
Tricep Stretch	p.117	
The Corkscrew	p.96	

Post-round rebalancing

Add the following exercises to those recommended for your postural type:

Spine Curls	p.45	
Hip Flexor Stretch	p.47	
Pelvic Stability	p.38	
Side Rolls	p.54	
Curl Ups	p.78	

Oblique Curl Ups	p.79	
Ankle Circles	p.44	
Cherry Picking	p.189	
Beach Ball Hamstring Stretch	p.123	
Working the Arches	p.74	
The Diamond Press or The Dart	p.110 or p.70	
Rest Position	p.73	
Arm Openings	p.52	

Angling and Sea Fishing

Statistically a sport more popular even than running or football, fishing can also take its toll on your body in several ways. Apart from the long hours spent either sitting on the bank or on rocks in the pouring rain or standing in cold water up to the thighs, there are injuries associated with casting – shoulder and elbow problems. Good casting technique will go a long way to preventing such problems but, in the meantime, while you are still working on the perfect action, try adding the following pre- or post-angling exercises to those recommended for your common postural type:

The Starfish	p.42	
Shoulder Drops	p.48	
Spine Curls	p.45	
Side Rolls	p.54	
Curl Ups	p.78	
Oblique Curl Ups	p.79	
The Diamond Press	p.110	

The Dart	p.70	
Rest Position	p.73	
The Corkscrew	p.96	
The Scapular Squeeze	p.134	
The Dumb Waiter	p.56	
Tricep Stretch	p.117	
Standing	p.56	
Standing Waist Twists	p.63	
The Arm Weight Series: Triceps	p.128	
Backstroke Swimming	p.126	
Roll Downs	p.68	
Arm Openings	p.52	

Swimming

Not only do we try to catch fish, we also try to emulate them! Swimming is without doubt one of the best and most enjoyable ways to keep fit. However, international and club swimmers alike suffer from a variety of problems directly related to their sport and, in particular, to their chosen stroke. Generally speaking, professional swimmers are liable to have problems related to their poor upper limb posture. They are often of the swayback postural type which is associated with overdeveloped rectus abdominis and obliques. These problems include:

- Over dominant latissimus dorsi
- An imbalance between the medial and external rotators of the shoulders
- Poor lumbar stability
- Overdeveloped rectus abdominis and obliques
- Muscle imbalances round the knee as they tend to rotate the knees
- Hyperextended legs
- Shoulder joint impingements
- Tight pectorals
- Over-dominant neck extensors
- Thoracic flexion

Try adding the following exercises to those recommended for your postural type:

The Starfish	p.42	
Windmill Arms	p.102	
Shoulder Drops	p.48	
The Diamond Press	p.110	
The Dart	p.70	
The Star	p.114	
Table Top with Sliding Legs	p.119	
Threading a Needle	p.77	
Rest Position	p.73	
The Corkscrew	p.96	
Single Leg Stretch or The Hundred or Double Leg Stretch	p.106 or p.120 or p.108	
Oblique Curl Ups or Oblique Single Leg Stretch	p.79 or p.163	
Hip Flexor Stretch	p.47	
Arm Openings	p.52	
Chalk Circle (unless you have a shoulder problem)	p.136	

Water Sports

Sailing

Sailors may have a variety of problems arising from being in a confined space and requiring considerable strength to sail the boat. Generally speaking, most sailors have a lack of flexibility from holding sustained positions for long periods of time, resulting in muscles becoming short and stiff. Sailors rarely do any cross training which compounds the problem.

Common problems are:

- The tucked position held while sailing often leads to over-dominant hip flexors and upper abdominals as you cling to the boat
- Forward-poking chin
- Thoracic flexion (rounded shoulders)
- Tight upper trapezius and levator scapulae as you use the tiller and winches
- Medially rotated shoulder girdles
- Protracted shoulder blades

Include the following exercises into the programme recommended for your postural type:

The Compass	p.31	
The Starfish	p.42	
Spine Curls	p.45	

Hip Flexor Stretch	p.47	
Side-lying Quadriceps and Hip Flexor Stretch	p.84	
The Diamond Press	p.110	
The Dart	p.70	
The Star	p.114	
Rest Position	p.73	
Single Leg Stretch or The Hundred or Double Leg Stretch	p.106 or p.120 or p.108	
The Arm Weight Series: Flys (but without weights)	p.125	
Floating Arms	p.58	
The Dumb Waiter	p.56	
Tricep Stretch	p.117	
Pole Raises	p.60	
The Scapular Squeeze	p.142	
Arm Openings	p.52	

Water Skiing

Water skiers often suffer trauma injuries as they hit the water, otherwise many of their problems arise from gripping the bar. An experienced skier will use his strong centre to bring him up out of the water, a beginner is more likely to pull on his arms instead.

Problems:

- Dominant pectorals
- Massive thoracic flexion (rounded shoulders)
- Nerve injuries in the forearms
- Irritable discs or facet joints
- Low back strain

Try adding these exercises to those recommended for your postural type:

Spine Curls	p.45	
Hip Flexor Stretch	p.47	
Curl Ups	p.78	
Oblique Curl Ups	p.79	
Arm Weights Series: Triceps	p.128	

Single Leg Stretch or The Hundred or Double Leg Stretch	p.106 or p.120 or p.108	
Oblique Single Leg Stretch	p.79	
Lying Side Stretch	p.116	
Side-lying Quadriceps and Hip Flexor Stretch	p.84	
Table Top with Sliding Legs	p.119	
The Diamond Press	p.110	
The Dart	p.70	
The Star	p.114	
The Dumb Waiter	p.56	
Pole Raises	p.60	
The Scapular Squeeze	p.142	
The Rest Position	p.73	
Arm Openings	p.52	

Rowing

Repetitive action in a sustained position in cramped conditions. Need we say more?

Rowers may have the following problems:

- Low back problems due to lack of lumbar stability
- Tight rectus abdominis
- Held thoracic flexion (rounded shoulders)
- Which leads to rib and shoulder problems
- Knee problems due to imbalance in the leg muscles and maltracking of the patella (knee cap)

Add the following to your training programme along with the exercises recommended for your postural type:

Roll Downs	p.68	
Pole Raises	p.60	
The Dumb Waiter	p.56	

Spine Curls	p.45	
Side Rolls	p.54	
Side-lying Quadriceps and Hip Flexor Stretch	p.84	
Curl Ups	p.78	
Oblique Curl Ups	p.79	
Single Leg Stretch or The Hundred or Double Leg Stretch	p.106 or p.120 or p.108	
Oblique Single Leg Stretch	p.79	
The Star	p.114	
The Dart	p.70	
Rest Position	p.73	
Table Top with Sliding Legs	p.119	
Up and Down with a Tennis Ball	p.88	

'Pilates is helping British Oarsmen prepare for Sydney 2000. Correct activation of deep postural abdominals supplements the action of the powerful low back muscles during the propulsion phase of the stroke. Improving Core Stability through Pilates is also reducing the incidence of low back pain resulting in a "healthy" population of oarsmen.'

Wendy Green MCSP, SRP, Grad Dip.
Physiotherapist Great Britain Rowing Squad
Body Control Pilates Instructor

Athletics

See also Running on page 217.

This is a huge subject as each track and field event results in its own imbalances and injuries. For the throwing events such as javelin and discus, for example, scapular stability work needs to be added. However, it is possible to add a set of exercises to the general training programmes because all events need trunk stability. In addition, all athletes will benefit from the lateral breathing techniques used in Body Control Pilates, which will greatly improve lung capacity and therefore oxygen intake. As the training regimes become more sophisticated and complex, a return to sound basics is essential.

Add the following exercises to your training programme and to those recommended for your postural type:

The Starfish	p.42	
Pelvic Stability	p.38	
Spine Curls	p.45	
Side-lying Quadriceps and Hip Flexor Stretch	p.84	
Curl Ups (watch out for dominating rectus and hip flexors)	p.78	
Oblique Curl Ups	p.79	
Hip Rolls	p.101	
Hamstring Stretch	p.82	

Adductor Stretch	p.80	
Single Leg Stretch or Double Leg Stretch	p.106 or p.108	
The Hundred	p.120	
Foot Exercises	p.74	
The Diamond Press	p.110	
The Dart	p.70	
The Rest Position (focus on breathing)	p.73	
Side Reaches	p.64	
Roll Downs	p.68	

For participants in throwing events, add these to those above:

Floating Arms	p.58	
The Dumb Waiter	p.56	
The Corkscrew	p.96	
Pole Raises	p.60	
Arm Openings and Chalk Circle, as long as there is no injury	p.52 and p.136	

Running

In this section we are looking at serious runners and joggers. Jogging is still one of the most popular ways to keep fit, yet it can be fraught with injury potential. One of the main problems is that the majority of running is done on pavements or on concrete and, as a result, joints throughout the body are repeatedly jarred and stressed. Add to this poor running style and existing muscle imbalance and you have all the right ingredients for problems. Poor running style is particularly common among long-distance runners, sprinters have to get their technique right or they'll get no further than the starting blocks!

As a general rule, most runners, whether long or short distance, have the following muscle imbalances:

- Over dominant quadriceps
- Over dominant hamstrings
- Long-distance runners have weak gluteals
- Poor pelvic stability
- Weak transversus abdominis
- Tight tensor fascia latae
- Medially rotated femurs
- Weak intrinsic foot muscles, poor arches (spend a fortune on the right running shoes but forget to work the muscles of the feet)
- 'Compartment syndrome' – many runners suffer from this condition which involves a build up of pressure in the lower limbs simply because of overuse
- Poor breathing patterns

We have suggested a few preparatory pre-run exercises, the second list should be included in your general training programme and added to those recommended for your postural type.

Pre-run Warm Up (15 minutes)

Lateral Breathing	p.29	
Roll Downs	p.68	
Side Reaches	p.64	
Pelvic Stability	p.38	
Spine Curls	p.45	
Side-lying Quadriceps and Hip Flexor Stretch	p.84	
Curl Ups	p.78	
Side Rolls or Hip Rolls	p.54 or p.101	
Hamstring Stretch	p.82	
Ankle Circles and Cherry Picking	p.44 or p.189	
Adductor Stretch	p.80	
The Dart	p.70	
Rest Position (unless you have knee problems)	p.73	

Add to your overall training:

The Starfish	p.42	
Knee Stirs	p.43	
Single Leg Stretch or Double Leg Stretch	p.106 or p.108	
The Hundred	p.120	
Standing on One Leg	p.94	

Table Top	p.118	
The Star	p.114	
The Diamond Press	p.110	
Rest Position (unless you have knee problems)	p.73	
Leg Weight Series: Twenty Lifts (to strengthen gluteus medius)	p.131	
Foot Exercises	p.74	

'I consider Body Control Pilates to be a very valuable adjunct in the prevention and rehabilitation of sports injuries and postural pain.'

Carol Russell MSc, MCSP, SRP
Body Control Pilates Instructor. Sportswise, Eastbourne. Chief Physiotherapist to Team England for the Commonwealth Games Kuala Lumpur 1998 and Manchester 2002

Skiing

How many skiing holidays end in plaster casts! We may not be able to lessen the risk of trauma injuries but, at the very least, we can make sure that your muscles are strong and flexible enough to cope with the enormous demands which this exhilarating sport makes on your body. Going straight from working in an office to the ski slopes is nothing short of foolhardy unless you prepare your body first.

You are going to need:

- Very strong quadriceps, especially vastus medialis
- Good pelvic stability so strong gluteus medius
- Strong deep lower abdominals, especially transversus abdominis and internal obliques
- Good scapular stability to help with using the ski poles
- Good ankle mobility – we need to strengthen the dorsi flexors
- Toe exercises to help the plantar fascia which gets really tight and overworked in ski boots
- Exercises to correct thoracic flexion
- Exercises to increase your proprioception

Before you set off skiing, add the following exercises to those recommended for your postural type:

Sliding Down the Wall	p.66	
Spine Curls	p.45	
Curl Ups	p.78	

Oblique Curl Ups	p.79	
The Diamond Press	p.110	
The Dart	p.70	
Rest Position	p.73	
Foot Exercises	p.74	
The Hundred	p.120	
Leg Weight Series: Passé Développés, Battement, Circles	p.170, p.172, p.173	
Hip Flexor Stretch	p.47	
Side-lying Leg Weights, especially twenty up and down in front	p.130	
Single Leg Stretch or The Hundred or Double Leg Stretch	p.106 or p.120 or p.108	
Side-lying Quadriceps and Hip Flexor Stretch	p.84	
Pole Raises	p.60	
Standing on One Leg	p.94	
The Scapular Squeeze	p.142	
Up and Down with Tennis Ball – try squeezing a pillow between the knees as you go up and down	p.88	
The Pillow Squeeze	p.86	

Cycling

'Pilates is to be strongly recommended for most athletes but in particular for cyclists, as their sport causes them to overuse their mobilizing muscles and underuse their deep stabilizing muscles. A healthy tree must have a strong trunk and roots to support and nourish its branches. If not, that tree will eventually topple or become malformed.

Compare this to an athlete's body . . . with Pilates, not only are the stabilizing muscles strengthened but also the respiratory, circulatory and lymphatic systems are stimulated to work more efficiently. In cycling, by strengthening the stabilizing muscles, the mobilizing muscles can function better and balance is restored, so optimizing a cyclist's performance and competitive capacity.'

Jan Van de Velde
Osteopath and physiotherapist to the Belgian Cycling Federation and the Belgian national cycling team; Osteopath for the professional Lotto Cycling Team; President of the Belgian Triathlon Federation; President of the Flemish Triathlon League.

Cycling is a healthy sport that enables you to become fit relatively quickly. However, it also involves holding an awkward position for sustained periods of time, which may then result in the following imbalances and problems:

- Dominant hip flexors
- Dominant hamstrings
- Dominant quadriceps
- Weak gluteals
- Overused ankle dorsiflexors (tight shins, which means that you lose the ability to point the foot)

- Shoulder protraction (rounded shoulders) as you grip the handle bars
- Tight pectorals and upper trapezius
- Forearm overuse injuries
- Upper limb nerve irritation
- Low back pain due to being flexed forward and the back and pelvis being rigid
- Hypermobile ankles

Try adding the following exercises to those recommended for your postural type:

The Compass	p.31	
Spine Curls	p.45	
Ankle Circles	p.44	
Hamstring Stretch	p.82	
Side-lying Quadriceps and Hip Flexor Stretch	p.84	
The Diamond Press	p.110	
The Dart	p.70	
The Star	p.114	
Rest Position	p.73	
Leg Weight Series: Twenty Lifts (to strengthen gluteus medius)	p.131	
Standing on One Leg	p.94	

Up and Down with a Tennis Ball	p.88	
The Dumb Waiter	p.56	
The Corkscrew	p.96	
The Cossack	p.62	
Triceps Stretch	p.128	

The Spine Stretch	p.124	
Foot Exercises	p.74	
Arm Openings	p.52	
Chalk Circle	p.136	

Equestrian Sports

There is no doubt that man and horse have a special affinity but, unfortunately, nature did not necessarily design our bodies with this relationship in mind! With horse riding, as with many of the other sports we have discussed, good technique is central not only to success but also to prevention of injury. Even with excellent technique, however, you are still liable to postural problems. A jockey will usually have rounded shoulders, with dressage you will tend to have dominant inner thighs, then there is always the added problem of falling off! Having said this, we can help to prevent these problems developing into anything more serious.

Generally speaking, equestrians across the board may suffer from:

- Over-dominant adductors (sometimes you can still see the shape of the horse!)
- Over-dominant hip flexors
- Spinal problems due to lack of lumbar stability. Good riders should use their gluteals to drive the horses forward but less experienced riders often tend to use their backs
- Weak abdominals
- Jockeys and hunters may be round shouldered
- Poor scapular stability
- Overlong Achilles tendons (from the foot position in the stirrups)

Add the following to those exercises recommended for your postural type:

Relaxation Position	p.28	
The Compass	p.31	
The Starfish	p.42	
Spine Curls	p.45	
Hip Flexor Stretch	p.47	
Curls Ups (when stronger Single Leg Stretch, The Hundred or Double Leg Stretch)	p.78, (106,129, 108)	
Oblique Curl Ups or Oblique Single Leg Stretch	p.79 or p.163	
Side-lying Quadriceps and Hip Flexor Stretch	p.84	
The Diamond Press or The Dart (jockeys and hunters do both)	p.110 or p.70	
Rest Position	p.73	
Foot Exercises	p.74	
Up and Down with a Tennis Ball	p.88	
Leg Weight Series, Twenty Lifts but not Adductor Lifts	p.130	
Adductor Stretch, then Wide Leg Stretch Against the Wall	p.80, p.81	
Threading a Needle	p.77	
Arm Openings or Chalk Circle	p.52 or p.136	

Jockeys and hunters add:

The Dumb Waiter	p.56	
The Corkscrew	p.96	
Pole Raises	p.60	

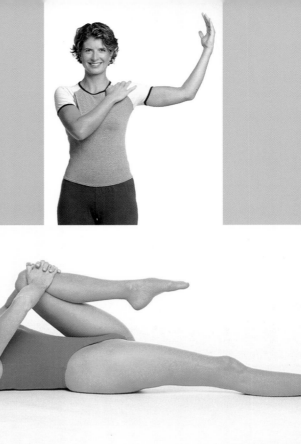

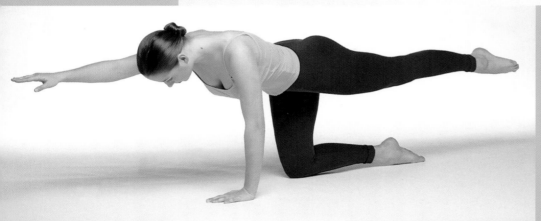

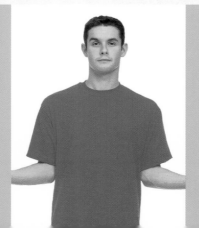

Body Control Pilates
and the
Performing Arts

For many years it was only performers who knew about Pilates! When Joseph Pilates opened his New York Studio in the 1920s, his early clients were from the ballet and acting communities. Today these groups need little convincing about the benefits of Pilates because they have seen the wonderful results on disciples who have been practising for many years.

'Pilates is a fundamental part of my dance training.'

Wayne Sleep

Actors

Pilates has long been popular among actors, particularly when they have a nude scene to play. The long lean look they are able to achieve means they don't need to use body doubles. On a more serious front, acting requires enormous stamina and endurance, enhanced body awareness, excellent body alignment and voice projection. All these can be greatly improved through Pilates.

Add the following exercises to those recommended for your postural type:

Standing Correctly	p.56	
Lateral Breathing	p.29	
Sliding Down the Wall	p.66	
Roll Downs	p.68	
Curl Ups	p.78	
Oblique Curl Ups	p.79	

Single Leg Stretch or The Hundred or Double Leg Stretch	p.106 or p.120 or p.108	
The Diamond Press	p.110	
The Dart	p.70	
Rest Position	p.73	
Side Rolls or Hip Rolls	p54 or p.101	
Standing Waist Twists	p.63	
Floating Arms	p.58	
The Corkscrew	p.96	
Arm Openings	p.52	
Chalk Circle	p.136	

'Pilates is the single most effective exercise technique I have ever known.'

Stephanie Powers

Dancers

Pilates exercises offer the perfect complement to traditional dance training. Very often dancers are expected to work at the end range of movement and with the legs turned out. It is very useful, therefore, to make them focus on exercises which keep the range within the 'box-shape' of the body, knees not wider than shoulder-width apart and legs in parallel. It is also important for them to build strength at the centre (proximally) and work from this rather than building strength peripherally (distally). Many of their injuries are a result of working long hours when tired and dancing on unsprung floors. Like many top sports people there is enormous pressure for dancers to carry on while injured, which can only exacerbate the problem. Common problems experienced by dancers:

- Overstretched muscles and nerves
- Ankle injuries, short Achilles tendons
- Foot injuries from working on points and landing from jumps
- Knee injuries from forcing them to turn out
- Neck problems from bad spotting
- Lower limb stress fractures
- Hyperextended knees
- Poor proprioception (this is surprising but often as result of taking everything to the extreme)
- Arthritis of the hips
- Amenorrhoea (lack of menstruation due to poor eating habits)
- Osteoporosis (for the above reason)

Try adding the following exercises to your usual training and to those recommended for your postural type. The swayback posture is very common among dancers as is the habit of posteriorly rotating the pelvis or tucking.

Relaxation Position – Compass	p.28 and p.31	
Spine Curls	p.45	
Knee Stirs with bent and/ or straight leg	p.43	
Ankle Circles	p.44	
Cherry Picking	p.189	
Curl Ups or, if more advanced, Single Leg Stretch or The Hundred or Double Leg Stretch	p.78, p.106, p.120, p.108	
Oblique Curl Ups or Single Leg Stretch	p.79 or p.106	
Foot Exercises	p.74	
The Dart then Dart into Side Bend	p.70, p.156	
Table Top	p.118	
Rest Position	p.73	
Floating Arms	p.58	
The Dumb Waiter	p.56	
Side Reaches	p.64	
Standing Waist Twists	p.63	
Arm Weight Series	pp.125 –9	
Chalk Circle	p.136	

Musicians

Sitting astride a cello, nestling a violin into your chin, holding a flute to your lips or sitting at a piano – any of the above will cause postural problems in the body because they involve holding sustained positions for hours on end.

Depending on your instrument you may find yourself suffering from:

- Medially rotated shoulders
- Overworked upper trapezius
- Weak scapular stabilizers
- Neck and forearm problems
- Thoracic flexion (rounded shoulders)
- Hand, wrist and finger problems

The following exercises should be done before or after you play to balance the body. You should also take time to do those exercises recommended for your postural type.

Roll Downs	p.68	
Spine Curls	p.45	
Hip Flexor Stretch (if you sit while you play)	p.47	
Curl Ups	p.78	
Oblique Curl Ups	p.79	
As you get stronger, add Single Leg Stretch or The Hundred or Double Leg Stretch	p.106 or p.120 or p.108	
The Diamond Press	p.110	
The Dart	p.70	
Rest Position (unless you have knee problems)	p.73	
The Cossack and Standing Waist Twist	pp.62–3	
Floating Arms	p.58	
The Dumb Waiter	p.56	
The Corkscrew	p.96	
Hand and Finger Exercises	p.229	

Hand and Finger Exercises

Starting Position
- Stand correctly, shoulder blades down into your back

Action
1 Hold your hands out in front of you, elbows soft.
2 Take the first and second fingers together away from the fourth and fifth fingers, creating a gap in the middle.
3 Return to centre.
4 Repeat eight times.

Action
1 Leaving the second and third fingers in the centre, take the first and fifth fingers away.
2 Return to centre.
3 Repeat eight times.

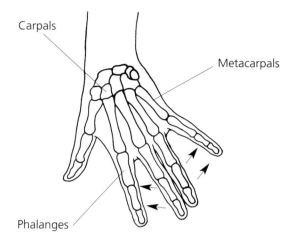

The bones of the hand

Carpals

Metacarpals

Phalanges

Singers

As a singer, you are going to need excellent breathing techniques and a strong centre. You will also find that the correct relationship between the head and neck can dramatically improve your voice. By improving your overall posture you will be able to stand at rehearsals and during performances for hours on end without tiredness.

Add the following exercises to those recommended for your postural type:

Relaxation Position	p.28	
The Starfish	p.42	
Neck Rolls	p.50	
Spine Curls	p.45	
Ankle Circles	p.44	
Cherry Picking	p.189	

Up and Down with a Tennis Ball	p.88	
Curl Ups or, if more advanced, Single Leg Stretch or Double Leg Stretch	p.78, or p.106, or p.108	
Oblique Curl Ups	p.79	
The Hundred	p.120	
The Diamond Press	p.110	
Rest Position (unless you have knee problems)	p.73	
Lumbar Stabilization	p.33	
The Dumb Waiter	p.56	
Chalk Circle	p.136	
Scarf Breathing	p.29	

'I distinctly remember after only one session with Gordon walking out feeling a different shape, centred, grounded, and happy! As an opera singer it's given me a strength I never knew I had – but then came the challenge – what could it do for a body after triplets?! The books are the answers to my prayers – at home and at work!'

Janis Kelly, Opera Singer

'I'd had enough of looking red and sweaty in a spandex leotard, so Pilates came as a relaxing, strengthening graceful relief. I'd started out as a muscley aerobicised 80s product, and ended up a slender, upright 90s swan – under Gordon's careful tutelage.'

Tracy Ullman

'It was my theatrical agent who first whispered the name Gordon Thomson to me: some new method which lengthened muscles rather than beefing them up, which pulled in the stomach and lengthened the spine. [Gordon] took me and my body in hand. It literally changed me day by day; there could be no mistake about it . . . I finally found my proper shape. There was no area of my life that didn't improve radically.'

Simon Callow

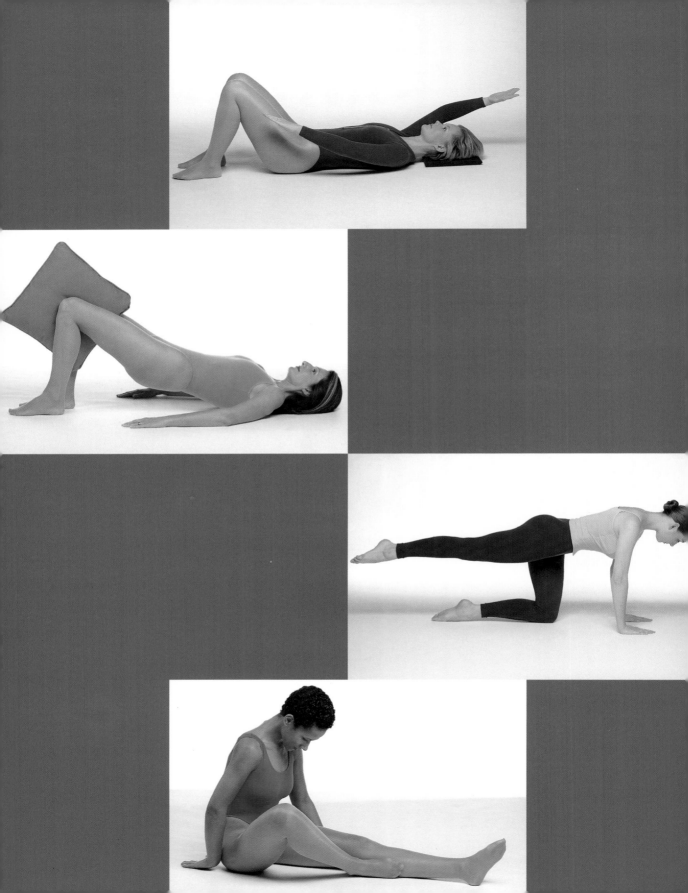

Body Control Pilates
for Health

Women's Health

In Body Control Pilates you have an exercise regime which can be adapted to whatever stage of life you are at. Not only will it help you to look your best throughout your life, but it can also help to prevent many of the health problems associated with being female!

Menstruation

We have put a short session together which we hope will help you should you be suffering from bad period pains.

Pelvic Clocks	p.100	
The Starfish	p.42	
Shoulder Drops	p.48	
Spine Curls (don't come up too high)	p.45	
Curl Ups (gentle)– keep the abdominal work very gentle as your transversus does not work as efficiently	p.78	
Chalk Circle	p.136	
Arm Openings	p.52	
Sliding Down the Wall	p.66	
Knee Stirs	p.43	
Adductor Stretch	p.80	

Also try this comforting exercise:

Knee Circling

Action

1 Lie in the Relaxation Position, zip up and hollow.
2 Bring your knees up towards your chest so that they are directly over your hips. Place your hands on each knee and very gently circle the knees in opposite directions.
3 Repeat ten times each way.

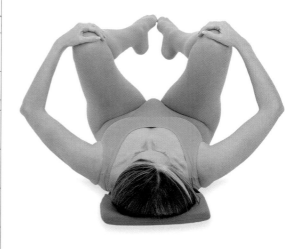

You should find this massages your low back – just check that you stay in neutral.

Preparing for Pregnancy

We strongly believe that you should prepare your body before you become pregnant so that it is in peak condition, thus providing the best possible start for yourself and your baby. Pilates will help ensure that everything is working as nature intended, that your pelvis and all your internal organs are correctly positioned and your respiratory, circulatory and lymphatic systems are efficient. Your abdominals and pelvic floor will need to be strong enough to support the 'bulge' yet not so strong that problems may occur (see below).

Add the following to those recommended for your postural type:

The Starfish	p.42	
Spine Curls with Pillow	p.98	
Hip Flexor Stretch	p.47	
Curl Ups (gentle)	p.78	
Oblique Curl Ups (gentle)	p.79	
Roll Downs	p.68	
The Corkscrew	p.96	
The Cossack	p.62	
The Diamond Press or The Dart	p.110 or p.70	
The Star	p.114	
Rest Position	p.73	

Pelvic Floor exercises: The Flower	p.237	
Arm Openings	p.52	

Ante-natal Exercises

Once you are pregnant it is very important that you adapt your fitness routine accordingly. You are not ill and there is no doubt that you and your baby will benefit enormously from exercise during this ante-natal period. You will, however, have to adapt your usual programme to take into account the changes taking place within your body. If you are doing any cardiovascular work in addition to Pilates, be careful not to raise your heart rate too high as you must remember that the foetal heart rate is already faster than your own.

The changes in the hormones results in ligamentous laxity. The ligaments (which join bone to bone) in the body soften to allow the pelvis to expand during the birth itself. This means that many of your joints may become unstable, in particular the sacroiliac joints. You will need to pay extra attention to alignment with every exercise you do. You will need good lumbar stability and pelvic alignment as the baby grows and puts extra strain on your back. The traditional stance of pregnancy with the hollowed back stresses the lumbar spine and you should try to be very body aware to avoid this.

Although good abdominal strength is necessary to support the spine this is not the time to work on over-strengthening these muscles or going for a flat stomach! The baby needs room to grow without restriction, so we recommend that abdominal work is limited to gentle transversus abdominis strengthening.

By working on your scapular stability, you will

lessen the effects of heavy breasts which can lead to rounded shoulders. The breathing techniques and overall body control will be very useful during labour as will good control of the pelvic floor muscles! A word about these. We want them to be efficient but not too strong – you must learn how to let them release during the actual birth itself – see the exercise called The Flower.

Avoid exercises which put any pressure on the pubic bone (pubic symphysis) which is liable to separate with the increased laxity of the ligaments. You may also find that exercises which involve lying on your back become uncomfortable from your third trimester onwards, so change position frequently. Working on all fours is a wonderful alternative and provides great relief as the pressure of the baby comes off the spine.

We recommend that you stop exercising completely between weeks 8 to 14 of the pregnancy as this is when you are most likely to miscarry and you should consult your practitioner before continuing with them.

Try the following exercises after due consultation with your medical practitioner. We have given you a good selection to chose from and remember, if you find lying on your back uncomfortable, change position immediately.

Standing Correctly	p.56	
Table Top	p.118	
Rest Position (you'll need to separate your knees to allow for bump room)	p.73	
Pelvic Stability	p.38	
Shoulder Drops	p.48	

Neck Rolls	p.50	
The Dumb Waiter	p.56	
Floating Arms	p.58	
The Corkscrew	p.96	
Pole Raises	p.60	
The Starfish	p.42	
Side Rolls (feet on the floor)	p.54	
Ankle Circles (good for reducing swelling)	p.44	
Cherry Picking	p.189	
Arm Openings (place a pillow between the knees and another wedged under the bump)	p.52	
Sitting Pelvic Floor Exercises: The Flower	p.237	
Passé Développés without weights	p.170	
Up and Down with a Tennis Ball	p.88	
Adductor Stretch	p.80	
The Pillow Squeeze	p.86	

For your pelvic floor work, try the Lumbar Stabilization exercise on page 33 but when you take the lift back down to the ground floor, don't stop there. Let it go completely down to the basement!

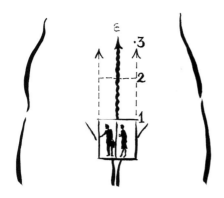

Another one for you . . .

Exercise: The Flower

Starting Position

- You may sit, stand or adopt The Relaxation Position for this exercise.

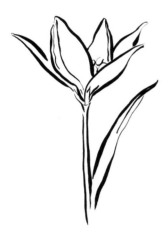

Action

1 Gradually draw the pelvic floor up and in just like a flower closing at the end of the day.
2 Now, gradually release the muscles, letting them open like a flower opening in the morning sun.

Post-natal exercises

Did you know that the test for continence requires you to be able to do ten Star Jumps on a full bladder. Any volunteers?

After the birth you are going to need a strong body to cope with the demands of motherhood. As the baby grows you will need to lift and carry, not just the baby, but all the paraphernalia that travels everywhere with you!

You must wait six weeks after the birth to have your final post-natal check-up before re-commencing exercise. We know that you want your figure back but if you attempt abdominal work too soon, you may do more harm than good. During your pregnancy the two halves of your rectus abdominis muscle will have separated to allow for the growth of the uterus. These two halves must rejoin (the midwife will do a 'rec test') before you begin Curl Up-style exercises or they may remain separated permanently. If you have had a Caesarean then you will need at least five months before you start Curl Ups. Zipping and hollowing is great to prepare you for this.

Pelvic floor exercises are the other areas to work. Lots and lots, please. Also exercises to strengthen the mid-back muscles, especially lower trapezius, otherwise the weight of your breasts as you breast-feed will stretch these muscles.

It will take several months for your hormones to return to normal so the ligaments will remain lax. Pay close attention to your alignment and do not try to overstretch. Do not introduce weights into your programme for at least six months and be careful of all exercises where you need good pelvic stability (such as standing on one leg) as your pelvis may still be unstable. The pelvic stability exercises in a lying position are fine as the floor supports you.

Be kind to yourself, take time out to relax, you will tire easily especially if you are breast feeding and getting little sleep. If you find lying on your front uncomfortable for your breasts, try the exercises on all fours instead.

Try the following exercises after six weeks in addition to those for your postural type:

Relaxation Position	p.28	
The Starfish	p.42	
Spine Curls with Pillow	p.98	
Hip Flexor Stretch	p.47	
Pelvic Stability	p.38	
Side Rolls	p.54	
Pelvic Floor exercises: Figure of Eight, The Emergency Stop	p.238, p.239	
The Star	p.114	
The Diamond Press	p.110	
The Big Squeeze	p.72	
Rest Position	p.73	
Roll Downs	p.68	
The Dumb Waiter	p.56	
Side Reaches	p.64	
Standing Waist Twists	p.63	

The Corkscrew	p.96	
Pole Raises	p.60	
Arm Openings	p.52	

In addition to the Lumbar Stabilization described on page 33, try the following:

Exercise: Figure of Eight

Starting Position
- Sit squarely on a chair, your feet hip-width apart and flat on the floor (use a cushion under them if necessary).
- Check that your pelvis is in neutral, your spine long and your shoulders relaxed.

Action
1 Take your awareness down to your pelvic floor.
2 Breathe out and try to close the urethra (from which you pass urine).
3 Breathe in and check that your shoulders are still relaxed.
4 Breathe out and, still lifting from the front, try to close the muscles round the anus (back passage) keeping your buttocks relaxed!
5 Breathe in, and double check that your shoulders and jaw are soft.
6 Breathe out, and add lifting from the vagina, holding all three openings.
7 Then slowly release.

Exercise: The Emergency Stop

Ever been caught short if you cough or sneeze? This is one to practice.

Action

1 Simply lift the whole of the pelvic floor, tightening it all quickly as if in an emergency. Hold for about five seconds, then release.
2 Practise five times.

Menopause

If you have been practising your Pilates regularly, when you do reach the menopause, you will reap the benefits a thousand fold. Your muscles will be toned so you can forget middle-aged spread. The work you have been doing with weights and resistance will help prevent osteoporosis (see page 253). Your joints will not stiffen and your body will remain supple and flexible. We have seen women in their sixties looking better than they did in their twenties because they have made a commitment to Pilates. And, if by chance you happen to be feeling a little irritable, lock yourself in a room with some peaceful music and exercise the mood out of your system. You can do this two ways, with de-stressing exercises such as Chalk Circle and Arm Openings or by working yourself really hard (place a pillow between the knees and then squeeze the life out of it!).

To keep you on the right track, add the following to the exercises recommended for your postural type:

Relaxation Position	p.28	
Shoulder Drops	p.48	
Spine Curls with Pillow	p.98	

Hip Flexor Stretch	p.47	
Pelvic Floor exercises: The Flower, Figure of Eight, The Emergency Stop	p.237, p.238, p.239	
Hip Rolls	p.101	
Curl Ups	p.78	
Oblique Curl Ups	p.79	
Hamstring Stretch	p.82	
The Big Squeeze	p.72	
The Diamond Press	p.110	
The Dart	p.70	
The Star	p.114	
Rest Position	p.73	
Roll Downs	p.68	
The Corkscrew	p.96	
The Leg Weight Series	pp.170 –3	
Arm Weight Series	pp.125 –9	
Adductor Stretch	p.180	
Up and Down with Tennis Ball	p.88	
Chalk Circle or Arm Openings	p.136 or p.52	

Men's Health

Having written so many pages on women's health, it seems only fair that we devote some space to men's health.

There are many ways in which Pilates can help improve men's health. Apart from all the general benefits which we have mentioned in the introduction and all the exercises devoted to individual sports activities, there are also specific health problems which Pilates exercises can help with.

All the pelvic floor exercises mentioned in the last chapter will be equally relevant for the prevention and treatment of prostate problems. If you zip up and hollow correctly you will be working your pelvic floor throughout the Pilates session.

Although Pilates is a non-aerobic exercise programme, this does not mean that the heart doesn't benefit from the sessions. Quite the opposite. The improvement in circulation is dramatic and, when the higher levels are attained, The Series of Five (page 174) will raise your heart rate. You should however plan extra cardiovascular work into your overall fitness regime.

For the stressed-out businessman, the relaxing nature of the sessions are very beneficial at the end of the day. If you find that you are addicted to the gym and using heavier weights, by practising Pilates alongside your gym workouts, your body at least has the chance to rebalance and you will be more aware of correct postural alignment and stability. And for the over sixties, if you have regularly practised your Pilates, your body will be more toned, more supple, more mobile – stronger and leaner than ever. What are you waiting for?

Add the following exercises to your regular workout and to those recommended for your postural type:

Relaxation Position	p.28	
Shoulder Drops	p.48	
Windmill Arms	p.102	
Hip Flexor Stretch	p.47	
Spine Curls	p.45	
Hip Rolls	p.101	
Hamstring Stretch	p.82	
Curl Ups	p.78	
Oblique Curl Ups	p.79	
Single Leg Stretch or The Hundred or Double Leg Stretch (when strong enough)	p.108 or p.120 or p.106	
Pelvic Floor Exercises: The Flower, Figure of Eight, The Emergency Stop	p.237, p.238, p.239	
The Dart	p.70	
The Big Squeeze	p.72	
Rest Position	p.73	
Roll Downs	p.68	
The Cossack and Standing Waist Twist	p.62	

Side Reaches	p.64		Arm and Leg Weight Series	pp.125–9 and pp.170–3	
Adductor Stretch	p.80		Arm Openings	p.52	

Body Control Pilates at School

Your school days may have once been the best days of your life but today's schoolchildren have enormous pressures placed on them mentally and physically. We would need to add another volume to discuss the emotional pressures.

It's a great pity that so few children walk to school as this is an excellent way to start and end the day. Instead they travel by train, bus or car which adds to the number of hours a day they spend sitting. Perhaps we should start a campaign to bring back those wonderful old Victorian sloped desks and schedules which had the teacher moving from classroom to classroom. The Victorian desks have been replaced with flat desks and small lockers and the timetable with one which means that the children have to carry their books round with them. We became optimistic briefly when carrying your backpack properly in the centre of your back hit the height of fashion, but the optimism was short lived as most schoolchildren still insisted on carrying their bags on one shoulder. The effect this has on the spine and the muscles of the trunk is horrendous.

Add to this the nightmare 'cool' stance of slumping and swaying back (to show off the freshly pierced navel) and it's no wonder we all develop postural problems.

There is also a great deal of stress placed on the more diligent teenagers around examination times. They need to take time out for themselves away from their books to relax and stretch.

We have to be realistic here – it's not easy to motivate teenagers to exercise. Fortunately teenage magazines are very responsible and most include a health and fitness page (usually sandwiched between the problem pages). What helps sell Pilates to the young is the impressive list of TV and film stars who swear by it. Pilates has always appealed to the rich, famous and glamorous. We are fortunate enough to include Leonardo di Caprio, Courteney Cox and several top sports stars among our devotees. That usually helps to convince them.

Add the following exercises to your fitness sessions:

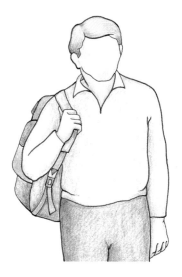 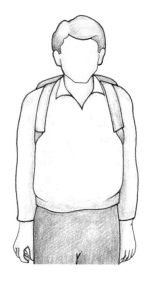

The Starfish	p.42	
Shoulder Drops	p.48	
Knee Stirs	p.43	
Spine Curls	p.45	
Hip Flexor Stretch	p.47	
Curl Ups (add Single Leg Stretch and DoubleLeg Stretch when they are ready)	p.78 (p.108, p.106)	
Oblique Curl Ups	p.79	
Side Rolls	p.54	

Roll Downs	p.68	
The Corkscrew	p.96	
Side Reach	p.64	
The Dart	p.70	
The Star	p.114	
The Rest Position	p.73	
Arm Openings or Chalk Circle	p.52 or p.136	

General Health

Back Problems

This is a huge topic and, when it comes to offering advice on exercise, is fraught with danger. Why? There are hundreds of different reasons why people have back pain and it is impossible to prescribe a remedial exercises programme without a proper diagnosis. Many causes of back pain will not be helped by exercise. We cannot stress strongly enough that you must seek medical advice before you embark on any exercise regime. Having said that, the majority of back problems are in fact caused by poor posture, muscle imbalances and misuse resulting in faulty movement patterns. Pilates exercises are perfect for these cases.

We have given you a selection of exercises which will help prevent back problems and which may be suitable in treating them. As a general rule, learn how to relax first, then add correct breathing techniques, then find your neutral alignment and do not move out of neutral until you can stabilize. Only add rotation and flexion on the advice of your consultant.

Add the following to the programme recommended for your postural type, taking into account the advice given above. Stop instantly if any movement causes you pain:

Relaxation Position	p.28	
The Starfish	p.42	
Pelvic Stability (avoid turning the leg out if you have sciatica)	p.38	
Shoulder Drops	p.48	

Neck Rolls	p.50	
Spine Curls	p.45	
Hip Flexor Stretch	p.47	
Curl Ups	p.78	
Oblique Curl Ups	p.79	
Floating Arms	p.58	
Pole Raises	p,60	
Side Reaches (if comfortable)	p.64	
The Diamond Press	p.110	
The Dart	p.70	
Rest Position	p.73	
Hamstring Stretch	p.82	
Adductor Stretch	p.80	
Ankle Circles	p.44	
Cherry Picking	p.189	
The Pillow Squeeze (can help certain types of sciatica)	p.88	

When you are stable you may add:

Side Rolls	p.54	
Standing Waist Twists	p.63	
Rolling Down the Wall	p.68	

The key to maintaining a healthy back lies not just in good exercise but in good movement and good posture whatever you are doing. Whenever you are standing, remember all your good standing directions (see page 56). You will find sound advice on how to sit at a desk on page 185. Take note also of the advice on driving on page 195. And on how to carry your backpack on page 242.

If you must relax in front of the TV at night, please avoid slumping, instead, maintain good posture and the natural curves of your spine, which, with a little care, is achievable even if you are sitting in an easy chair!

Even relaxing in an easy chair:

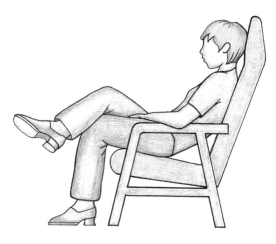

Avoid slouching

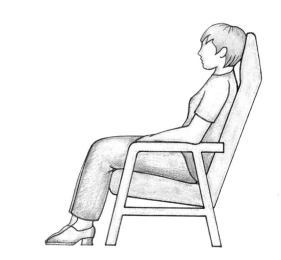

Sit as tall as possible

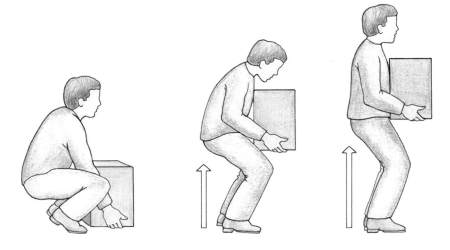

Lifting

When you lift a heavy object follow these guidelines:

- Stand close to the weight to be lifted
- Keep your back as straight as possible
- Face the object square on, not twisting
- Bend your knees to go down
- Hold the weight close to you.

As you lift the object, stabilize, and keep your back straight. Lift by straightening the knees. Try not to twist at all. If you have to turn, move your feet rather than your back.

Are you sleeping comfortably? It is a fallacy that your bed should be rock hard – it should be firm enough to support your spine when lying either on your back or on your side. Notice the pillows, they

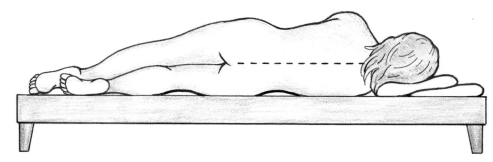

The spine is properly supported

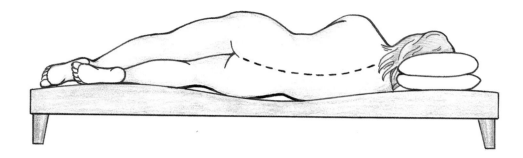

Here the spine sinks into the bed and the neck is at an awkward angle

should support the nape of your neck without allowing your head to tilt awkwardly or be pushed up out of good alignment.

Scoliosis

A scoliosis is a curvature of the spine with a lateral curve one way and a rotation the other. C-shape spines are often referred to as scoliosis, but they are in fact 'lists'.

The very nature of scoliosis is such that a general prescription is meaningless as every individual's curve will differ and requires specialist diagnosis. However, the overall lengthening, stability and breathing exercises contained in this programme could be beneficial:

Relaxation Position	p.28	
Lateral Breathing	p.29	
Lumbar Stability	p.33	
Spine Curls	p.45	
Sliding Down the Wall	p.66	
The Corkscrew	p.96	
Pole Raises	p.60	
The Diamond Press	p.110	
The Star	p.114	
The Dart	p.70	
Rest Position	p.73	
Roll Downs	p.68	

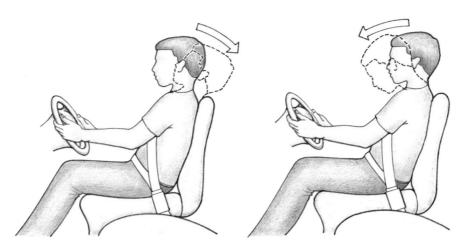

Whiplash and Other Neck Problems

We tend to think of whiplash injuries in association with car accidents, but they are also common as a result of contact sports such as rugby. With a whiplash injury the head is usually thrown violently forward, then backward and forward, which over-stretches and stresses the ligaments and which may result in such problems as ligament bleeds and facet joint and neural tissue damage. Any trauma to the neck will require immediate medical attention and follow-up specialist treatment to allow time for the inflammation to settle and the ligaments to heal.

Exercise does have a role to play but much later in the rehabilitation programme and only on the advice of the practitioner. When that time comes, Pilates is ideal because its gentle pace and slow, controlled movements mean that you can work isolated parts of the body without stressing the neck at all. Sometimes a cervical roll is useful to support the neck.

Generally speaking, bearing in mind that each case is different, we recommend that you avoid all flexion of the neck, which means you keep the head down on the mat – no curling up from the floor (you can still work the abdominals with pelvic stability exercises and abdominal hollowing). Neck

Rolls may aggravate the condition; Roll Downs would be contra-indicated as well; you may find that raising the arm causes pain. Some exercises can be adapted, for example in The Starfish the arm can be moved to the side rather than overhead. This still establishes a movement pattern. Neural tissue is sensitive so that stretches to other parts of the body can aggravate the problem so take care, move slowly and stop if in discomfort. You will probably find that many intermediate and advanced exercises are not suitable.

The following exercises may be included after consultation with your practitioner:

Relaxation Position (use a cervical roll if this helps)	p.28	
Lateral Breathing	p.29	
Lumbar Stabilization (Sitting)	p.33	
Pelvic Stability Exercises: The Flower, Figure of Eight, The Emergency Stop	p.237, p.238, p.239	
Side Rolls (keep your head in the centre)	p.54	
Hip Flexor Stretch	p.47	

Hamstring Stretch (take care with this one, see note on stretching above)	p.82	
Standing Correctly	p.56	
Sliding Down the Wall	p.66	
Up and Down with a Tennis Ball	p.88	
The Dumb Waiter	p.56	
The Diamond Press	p.110	
The Dart (keep your head down and simply engage the muscles under the shoulder blades)	p.70	
The Big Squeeze	p.72	
Table Top with Leg Sliding – no arms	p.119	
The Pillow Squeeze	p.86	

Please also note the good advice given under back problems about sleeping (page 246) and also the guidelines on how to sit at a desk on page 185, how to drive on page 195, how to carry your backpack on page 242 and finally how to use the telephone on page 185.

Foot Problems

Why are foot exercises so important? If you compare your body to a house, the feet would be the foundations of the building. You would not build a house on poor foundations, would you?

When evolution 'designed' the foot, it expected us to be romping through fields, climbing over rocks and stony ground, gripping slippery surfaces. All this action would have given the feet a natural workout, keeping them strong and flexible. Every reflexology point on the base of the feet would have been naturally massaged by the ground, so stimulating the rest of the body.

What do we have to offer our feet today? Fourteen hours plus cramped in the same shoes, walking on flat, even pavements. It is no substitute. Even when we take part in sport, we often forget the feet. Once we've chosen the right training shoes for the sport, we assume that's enough, but can you imagine putting your hands in a shoe-like glove and then ignoring them all day?

But look at what the feet do for us! They are our contact point with the earth. They bear the entire weight of our bodies. They really are the foundations upon which our bodies are built. And, like all foundations, they need to be stable, to be able to bear our weight in a balanced way. Muscles remember long-accustomed habits, regardless of whether they are good or bad. If we can get our feet right, then the knees, upper legs, hips, pelvis and more will be in better alignment.

Don't forget that when we give you instructions for standing correctly, we start with the feet. Mentally draw two triangles from the base of the big toes, to the base of the small toes to the centre of the heels. You need to ground yourself on those two triangles with the weight evenly centred on them.

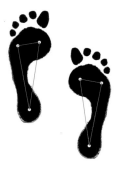

Flat Feet

Flat feet can change your whole postural stance, shortening the Achilles tendon and causing both upper- and lower-back imbalance. If the arches are weak, it will also contribute to the habit of rolling in the inside of the foot upsetting the foundations on which good posture are built. The arches are the shock absorbers of the feet – they literally put the spring in our step!

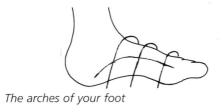

The arches of your foot

Keep your arches in shape with Working The Arches on page 74 and Cherry Picking on page 189.

If you allow the feet to roll in or roll out, you have upset your balance and your posture will be affected.

You can easily tell if you are prone to rolling in or out by checking your shoes: have they worn more on the outside or the inside of the heel? Similarly, you can easily spot if you put your weight more on the front or the back of your foot, as the toes of the shoes will curl up or the heels will be worn down in excess.

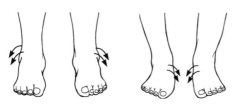

Rolling feet

The exercise on page 88 – Up and Down with a Tennis Ball is perfect for teaching good foot alignment.

The Toes and Joints

How can you become an expert in Body Control Pilates and have parts of your body totally outside your control? Get those toes moving . . . if nothing else, you'll be able to dry your nail varnish quicker!

Try The Mexican Wave on page 75.

Healthy Hips

Hip replacements are becoming close to an epidemic in modern society. You may blame our sedentary lifestyles and walking on hard flat pavements (which stresses the joint) but the greatest shame lies with the simple fact that the right exercises can help prevent the problem.

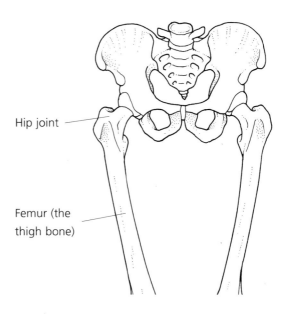

Hip joint

Femur (the thigh bone)

Pelvis and the thigh bone

The hip joint is a wonderful ball and socket joint, the head of the femur articulating freely in the hip socket the acetabulum, with a wide range of movement potential: flexion, extension, abduction, adduction, internal and external rotation circumduction. Yet during our normal everyday activities we tend to use just a fraction of this potential. For a joint to be healthy it needs to be taken regularly through its full range of movement to encourage the production of synovial fluid which lubricates the joint keeping it nourished and well oiled. The muscles round the joint need to be perfectly balanced so that the joint is in its neutral zone. These muscles will also need to be strong enough to support the joint itself.

If you have hip problems or have had a replacement you will need to consult your practitioner as some of the exercises below may not be suitable for your condition.

To help prevent hip problems and as a treatment for some hip problems (see above) try adding the following exercises to those recommended for your postural type:

Standing Correctly (in Floating Shoulders)	p.56	
Pelvic Stability Exercises	p.38	
Knee Stirs	p.43	
Passé Développés	p.170	
Leg Weight Series (abduction and adduction)	pp.170 –3	

In addition try this wonderful exercise which takes the head of the femur gently through internal and external rotation.

Exercise: Zigzags

Aim
To mobilize the hips, the knees and the ankle joints.

Starting Position
- Lie on the floor about half a metre away from a clear wall space. Your hips should be square to the wall, your head resting on a small flat pillow. Place the feet together on the wall.
- Check that your pelvis is in neutral.

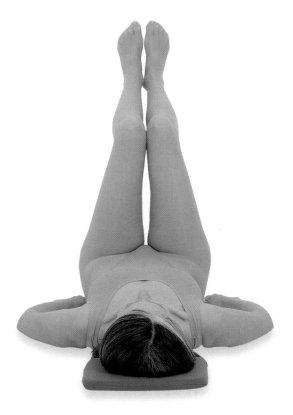

Starting position

Action

1 Slide your toes apart as far as they go, keeping the heels together.

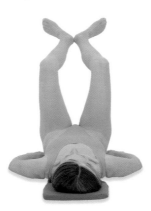

2 Now, keeping the balls of the feet still, slide the heels apart as far as they go.

3 Continue zigzagging the feet in this way, making certain that they stay flat on the wall.

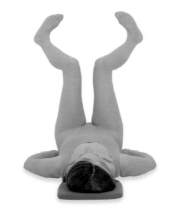

4 You should be transferring the weight of the feet alternately through the heels and through the balls of the feet.

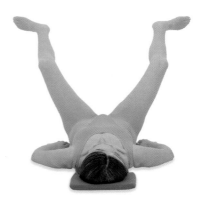

5 Zigzag until the feet refuse to turn any more. The legs are as wide as you can comfortably open them, without changing your pelvic alignment. Then zigzag back together again.

Watchpoints

- Check to see that the level of your feet has not dropped and that both feet are at the same height.
- Please try not to lift the feet off the wall. You are pivoting alternately on the balls and heels but letting the feet slide.
- Keep neutral!

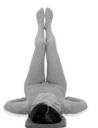 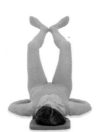 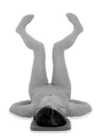 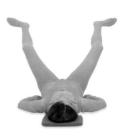

1. Starting position   *2.*   *3.*   *4.*

Osteoporosis

About 30 per cent of women and 5 per cent of men will suffer from osteoporosis or brittle bone disease. Osteoporosis is defined as a loss of bone mineral leading to thinning of the bone.

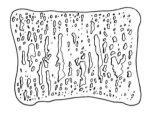

Healthy bone

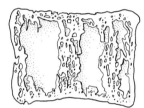

Brittle bone

Bone health is determined by nutrition, mineral and vitamin content and also by the amount of stress the bone is put under. This is one type of stress that is good for us because bones become thicker and stronger when they are stressed. This produces electrical effects in the bone which in turn encourages bone growth. If there is no stress, the bone will be less dense and weaker. During our lives there is a constant turnover of bone – up until the age of thirty-five we lose as much old bone each year as we make new bone so there is no problem. From then on we tend to lose about 1 per cent of our bone mass each year until we reach menopause, when bone loss accelerates with a further loss of 2 per cent per year for up to ten years. By the age of about seventy one third of bone mass will be lost – no wonder granny is shrinking!

Although bone looks very solid it is, in fact, full of holes rather like coral. We have two types of bone, trabecular bone which accounts for 20 per cent of our bone mass and cortical bone which accounts for the other 80 per cent. Trabecular bone is found mainly in the spine, pelvis and at the ends of long bones such as the head of the thigh bone. This is the bone which suffers most from a loss of density after the menopause. Cortical bone is found in the shafts of the long bones and the skull and here bone loss is more gradual. Most fractures which occur through osteoporosis occur at the wrist, the spine and the hip.

Bone mass is affected by:

- Hormonal status: menopausal women in particular have an accelerated bone loss, which comes with the decline of the production of the ovarian hormone, oestrogen.
- Dietary intake: especially the inclusion of naturally occurring plant oestrogens and calcium in our diet during our growing years.
- Genetic factors which determine the size of our bones and muscles.
- Physical activity, particularly weight-bearing exercise.

Recent research has shown that regular weight-bearing exercise can help prevent the onset of osteoporosis and the earlier we start weight training the better, even in our teens, as we are then laying good foundations for the future.

Many of our exercises use light hand and leg weights and are perfect for prevention of brittle bones. If you already have osteoporosis, you will need to consult your practitioner as the exercises may not be suitable for your condition. **As a general rule, it is wise to avoid all exercises which involve flexing the body (bending forward) as this will further encourage the hunched over** posture associated with osteoporosis, so avoid Curl Ups (and any exercises which involve lifting the head from the floor), Roll Downs, The Seal and Open Leg Rocker. Instead you should promote lengthening of the spine and correction of the back rounding forwards so gentle extension of the back is indicated, so practise The Diamond Press and The Dart.

The following Pilates exercises can be done using weights:

Leg Weights: Abductor Lifts	p.130	
Adductor Lifts	p.132	
Passé Développés (leave the head down on the mat)	p.170	
Arm Weights: Flys	p.125	
Backstroke Swimming	p.126	
Triceps	p.128	
Biceps	p.129	

Try the exercises first without weights, then start with a very light weight and work upwards. For the hand weights, start with 0.5 kilograms each weight and work up to 1.5 kilograms. The leg weights should be between 0.5 and 1.5 kilograms each weight.

If you have no weights, you can make your own hand weights by using a 100 gram can of beans or bag of rice, then 150 gram, 200 gram and so on. If you don't have a set of leg weights, take an old, clean pair of thick tights. Cut the legs off and about 15 centimetres from the toes tie a knot. Then weigh out between 0.5 and 1.0 kilograms of uncooked rice and pour it into the tights. Tie another knot about 20 centimetres away from the first knot. Now you have a set of weights which you can tie onto your ankles. A word of caution: pick a pair of tights with no holes or all the rice trickles through!

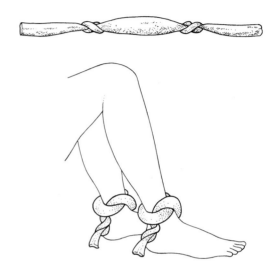

Making the weights

The following exercises can help to prevent osteoporosis and may be helpful in its treatment after due consultation with your practitioner:

Sliding Down the Wall	p.66	
The Starfish	p.42	
Spine Curls (take care if you have osteoporosis in the spine)	p.45	
Knee Stirs	p.43	
Knee Drops (in Pelvic Stability)	p.39	

Knee Folds	p.39	
Shoulder Drops	p.48	
The Arm Weight Series	pp.125 –9	
Leg Weight Series	pp.170 –3	
The Diamond Press	p.110	
The Dart	p.70	
The Big Squeeze	p.72	
Rest Position	p.73	
Pole Raises	p.60	
Arm Openings	p.52	

You could also try The Wrist Worker.

Exercise: The Wrist Worker

Aim

To strengthen the hands, wrists, forearms and upper arms while maintaining good posture.

It looks easy but this one is deceptive, as you really do work the whole arm. Please take advice if you are prone to tennis or golfer's elbow

Equipment

You'll need to make the worker itself. It's very simple. Take a 40 to 50 centimetre piece of dowel (wooden pole) which is about 2.5 centimetres in diameter. Drill a hole through the centre and thread

through a piece of rope which is about 1.5 metres long, tying a knot so that it is firmly secured.

To the other end of the rope you can attach a weight. You could use an old pair of tights or socks (clean) or a bag . Fill the bag with beans (dried, not baked) or rice or you could buy a bean bag. The weight can be between 0.5 to 1.5 kilograms.

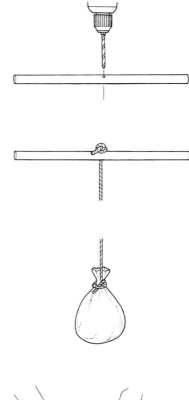

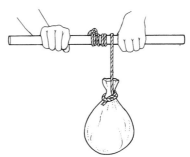

Steps to make the wrist worker

Starting Position

- The idea is that you start with the rope fully wound round the stick, then slowly unwind it fully before winding it up again.
- Stand correctly remembering all the directions given on page 56.
- Hold the wrist worker out in front of you, shoulder height, with your arms straight but not locked, parallel to the floor. Your hands should be placed on either side of the rope, holding underneath, with the palms up.
- You will breathe normally throughout.

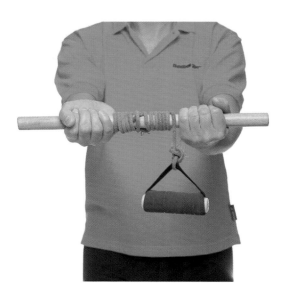

Action

1 Before you begin, lengthen up through the spine and zip up and hollow.

2 Make the wrist work, as you unravel the rope by moving one wrist downwards, the stick rotates towards you. The other hand will allow the stick to circle. Alternate wrists. Make sure that your shoulder blades stay down into your back and your neck and upper shoulders stay soft and relaxed.

3 When fully unravelled, change the hand position so that you are holding from above with the palms facing down as you roll the rope back up again. This time the stick rotates away from you.

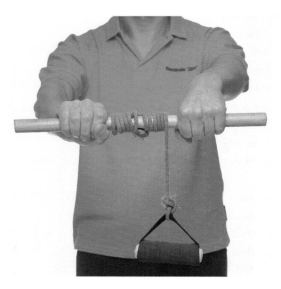

4 Once is enough for this exercise. When it becomes easier you may place a heavier weight in the bag.

5 To recap: palms facing up as the rope unwinds down; palms face down as the rope winds back up.

Watchpoints

- Don't let the shoulders creep up round your ears. Keep them soft and down.
- Keep your arms straight out in front of you. Don't let them drop.
- Don't skimp on the wrist movement. Make a full turn.

Osteoarthritis

This is most commonly due to wear and tear of the cartilage covering the ends of weight-bearing bones. As the cartilage starts to break up, the body produces new bone (osteophytes) in an attempt to prevent more wear and tear. It is easy to see, therefore, why athletes and dancers, in particular, are prone to arthritis through over use of joints such as the knee, hip and ankle. However, anyone is at risk if their joints are not in good alignment, as forces will stress the joint unevenly increasing the wear and tear. A good comparison would be the increase in wear on tyres where the wheels are not balanced evenly!

How can Pilates help? In lots of ways:

- For a joint to be healthy it needs to be taken regularly through its full range of movement, thus encouraging the production of synovial fluid to lubricate the joint keeping it nourished and well oiled. Body Control Pilates exercises gently take the joints through their full range of motion without placing the joint under any strain.
- With Pilates, you are always paying close atten-tion to the alignment of the body. This is crucial to the health of your joints for it encourages them to be in their neutral zone minimizing unwanted stress.
- Pilates strengthens the muscles round the joints, providing natural 'scaffolding' to support the joint and off-load unwanted forces.
- By working the stabilizing muscles of each joint, there is less shearing and therefore less wear and tear.

The beauty of Body Control Pilates is that it encour-ages natural movement in the body, restoring good alignment and rebalancing muscles. As a result you begin to move correctly all the time not just while you exercise – which means you will have far less wear and tear on all your joints.

As a general rule, you will want to mobilize your joints gently. Do not overstretch or take your joints out of their neutral zones. Avoid the use of weights.

The following exercises will help prevent osteoarthritis. If you already have osteoarthritis then you will need to consult your practitioner as some of the exercises may not be suitable for your condition:

The Starfish	p.42	
Knee Stirs	p.43	
Ankle Circles on the Wall	p.133	
Windmill Arms	p.102	
Spine Curls	p.45	
Pelvic Stability Exercises	p.38	
Side Rolls	p.54	
The Diamond Press	p.110	
The Dart	p.70	
Rest Position	p.73	
Sliding Down the Wall	p.66	
Floating Arms	p.58	
Passé Développés (no weights)	p.170	
Arm Openings	p.52	

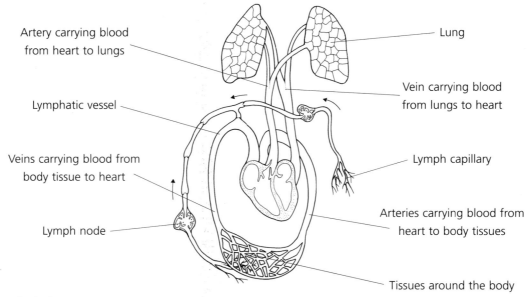

Artery carrying blood from heart to lungs

Lung

Vein carrying blood from lungs to heart

Lymphatic vessel

Veins carrying blood from body tissue to heart

Lymph capillary

Lymph node

Arteries carrying blood from heart to body tissues

Tissues around the body

Lymphatic System

Boost your Immune System

Joseph Pilates was very proud of the fact that none of his 'disciples' interned with him during the First World War died as a result of the flu epidemic which claimed the lives of millions worldwide. It is well known that exercise is good for boosting the immune system, and inducing the feel-good factor now known to have an impact on our overall health.

The Pilates Method is especially beneficial because it works on the respiratory, circulatory and lymphatic systems ensuring a better supply of nutrients and elimination of toxins right down at cell level. It is gentle enough to be used by all ages and levels of fitness and yet it is effective enough that you notice the difference immediately. It stands to reason that when you start to bring your body into good alignment, balancing the muscles and strengthening the core that your body will function more efficiently. All your internal organs will be

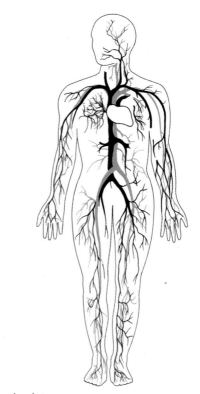

The circulatory system